Acute Toxicity
in
Theory and Practice

MONOGRAPHS IN TOXICOLOGY: ENVIRONMENTAL AND SAFETY ASPECTS

Edited by

J.W. Bridges

Institute of Industrial and Environmental Health and Safety, University of Surrey, Guildford, Surrey

and

P. Grasso

Medical Department, Occupational Health Unit, BP Research Centre, Sunbury-on-Thames, Middlesex

Acute Toxicity in Theory and Practice: With Special Reference to the Toxicology of Pesticides

V. K. Brown

Acute Toxicity
in
Theory and Practice

With Special Reference to the Toxicology of Pesticides

V. K. Brown

Shell Research Limited, Shell Toxicology Laboratory (Tunstall),
Sittingbourne Research Centre, Kent

A Wiley–Interscience Publication

JOHN WILEY & SONS

Chichester · New York · Brisbane · Toronto

British Library Cataloguing in Publication Data:

Brown, V.K.
  Acute toxicity in theory and practice.—
  (Monographs in toxicology, environmental and
  safety aspects).
  1. Pesticides—Toxicology
  I. Title II. Series
  632′.95042   RA1270.P4   79-42905

  ISBN 0 471 27690 1

Typeset by Preface Ltd., Salisbury, Wilts and printed
by Page Bros. (Norwich) Ltd., Norwich

Acknowledgements

The author gratefully acknowledges the generosity of Shell Research Limited in their support for the publication of this text. The advice of many colleagues within the Shell Group of Companies has been invaluable and, in particular, the editorial advice of Mr W. Pohl must be singled out for special mention. The burden of typing the draft manuscripts for this book has rested with Mesdames Janet Churchyard, Beryl Pilcher, and Rene Green, all of Shell Research Limited, Sittingbourne Research Centre, their dedication to detail and their helpful approach made completion of the book possible.

A suggestion by the author that this monograph should be written was enthusiastically encouraged by Professors J. W. Bridges, D. E. Stevenson, and A. N. Worden. Dr P. Grasso and Professor J. W. Bridges (editors of this series of books on environmental toxicology) and the publishers, John Wiley and Sons Limited, have been unfailingly helpful to the author. To all of these people and many others too numerous to name, many thanks.

Preface

When the author undertook the writing of this monograph there were three readerships in mind:

Firstly, students of toxicology, whether undergraduate or postgraduate, in Universities or Colleges together with those many people actively interested in the study of toxicology although not perhaps undertaking academic studies in the formal sense. This group of readers should not be put off by the deliberate emphasis on the toxicology of pesticides. This book is orientated towards the general principles of acute toxicology while utilizing the fact that the diverse properties of pesticides provide a plethora of examples to illustrate these principles.

Secondly, people in scientific administration. In particular the subject matter of the monograph should be of interest to those with a responsibility for creating legislation and those charged with administering the rules, regulations, and laws involving toxicology.

Thirdly, those people associated with the research, development, and ultimate use of pesticides. Some, possibly a minority, may feel uncertain about the real importance of acute toxicology in relation to their products and the importance of safety may be considered by some to be subjugated to the need to find a way of circumventing what may appear to be unnecessary legislative restrictions.

It is hoped that this monograph will provide some guidance for those concerned with the above activities and possibly others as well. It may be used as an introduction to the subject of even to reinforce background knowledge of the underlying principles of acute toxicology. If these objectives are met then the effort expended in writing this monograph will have been worthwhile.

Contents

Preface vii

Introduction 1

1 Prologue—justification of the need for acute toxicity information
for pesticides 6

2 Responses 14

3 Test animals 33

4 Dose and dosage 68

5 Exposure as a hazard and the various routes of exposure 81

6 The acute toxicology of pesticides in perspective 114

References 121

Index 156

Introduction

Too many acute toxicity tests are carried out on vertebrate animals in research on the development of commercial pesticides with little regard for the rationale of the investigation that has been undertaken. Sometimes this can be attributed to the naïve requirements of regulatory authorities but often it is the failure of the experimenter to appreciate the subject that gives rise to this wasteful situation. This book contains an analysis of some of the vast published literature appropriate to the acute toxicology of pesticides together with relevant details of some experimental procedures that may be used to elucidate some of the many problems associated with predictive acute toxicology testing.

It is necessary to establish some definitions that are applied throughout the text:

THE DEFINITION OF TOXICITY

Toxicity fits the criteria of a concept (Wilson, 1966) and an analysis of some of the ways by which this type of conceptual data can be utilized in risk assessment has been presented by Lowrance (1976); however it was Barnes (1963) who succinctly defined the toxicity of a product as its capacity to cause injury while the hazard attributable to a product represents the probability that it will do so. Barnes's definition is considered to be fundamentally correct and is the definition accepted by the National Academy of Sciences in the U.S.A. (Oser, 1971) and is used throughout this book. Hazard ranking is a very difficult process in which acute toxicity is but one factor (Jones, 1978).

THE DEFINITION OF ACUTE

The most relevant definition of acute in the Oxford English Dictionary is 'Coming sharply to a crisis, opposite to chronic' but this definition is linked, in the dictionary, to disease processes. To the toxicologist the term 'acute' can be used to define either the exposure or the response to an exposure, although the former is by far the more common connotation.

The most common use of the term acute in toxicology relates to exposure on one occasion only (i.e. single exposure). However, the term acute is sometimes considered acceptable for multiple exposures during a short period of time (Hagan, 1959), The period set for multiple exposures to be defined as acute is not clearly defined but a limit of within 24 hours is most generally acceptable.

Occasionally the term acute is also used to define the response and not the exposure.

THE DEFINITION OF PESTICIDE

According to the Oxford English Dictionary a pest is described as 'a troublesome or destructive animal or thing' and the suffix -cide implies 'slayer of or slaughter of'. Thus a pesticide is a product that kills animals, plants or micro-organisms that are troublesome or destructive.

A succinct definition of pesticide has been provided by the World Health Organization (Wld. Hlth. Org., 1976, Tech. Rept. Ser. No. 592): 'A pesticide is any substance or mixture of substances intended for preventing or controlling any unwanted species of plants and animals and also includes any substances or mixture of substances intended for use as a plant–growth regulator, defoliant or desiccant. The term "pesticide" includes any substance used for the control of pests during the production, storage, transport, marketing or processing of food for man or animals or which may be administered to animals for the control of insects or arachnids in or on their bodies. It does not apply to antibiotics or other chemicals administered to animals for other purposes, such as to stimulate their growth or to modify their reproductive behaviour; nor does it apply to fertilizers.'

There are several definitions and detailed categorizations of the different types of pesticides available and these are generally attributable to the official organizations such as the U.S. Environmental Protection Agency and the World Health Organization but may be taken as being universal. As far as possible the International Organization for Standardization nomenclature for pesticides (*Bull. Wld. Hlth. Org.*, 1973, **49**, 169–204) has been used throughout this account for the names of products.

As long ago as the sixteenth century, Paracelsus (1493–1541) the Swiss philosopher, physician (unqualified), and lecturer in medicine wrote that 'All substances are poisons; there is none which is not a poison. The right dose differentiates a poison and a remedy'. It is a truism that any chemical entering the body must produce an effect or effects and these may be:

(i) *Beneficial*. Nutritional and therapeutic effects may alter the course of life in an advantageous manner.
(ii) *Physiological or adaptive*. The effect causes no apparent alteration in the course of life but the chemical may have helped maintain the accepted physiological status of the organism.
(iii) *Harmful*. These effects are the converse of beneficial causing a change in the course of the life in an adverse sense.

It is within the framework of harmful (iii) that the term toxic is most commonly used. However, despite the gradation of these responses, it is common practice in experimental toxicology to quantify the acute response or the response to an acute exposure in a quantal form thus investigating effects in statistical populations rather than investigating individual responses (Wilks, 1971).

Although it is by no means the only toxic phenomenon observed, the most commonly measured response in investigations of acute toxicity is death (Hunter and Smeets, 1976). It is necessary to establish what is meant by life and by death in this context:

(a) *Life*. Life may be considered as being a stochastic process (Sacher and Trucco, 1962; Benjamin and Haycocks, 1970); thus two things are implied, an ordered sequence and a probability function generating the sequence. The alternative philosophy that life is a deterministic process (i.e. a stochastic process with a zero error of prediction) requires that the past completely determines the future of the system and that the system contains no random elements. It may be rationalized that life is a non-deterministic stochastic process and that the effects of toxicants are such that they alter the ordered sequence in an adverse sense and this change the probability function generating the sequence.

(b) *Death*. Death is the cessation of vital processes of the organism, that is the end-point of life. Because of the absolute form of death (i.e. within the context there is no gradation, the organism is either alive or it is dead) it is a convenient, discrete and finite end-point for use in quantal toxicometrics (Chapter 3).

Although toxicity and hazard have distinct meanings (Barnes, 1963), it is common for the measured toxicity to be used in hazard assessment. It has been suggested that safety can be expressed as the inverse function of the product of toxicity and bioavailability:

$$\text{Safety} \propto \frac{1}{(\text{Toxicity} \times \text{Bioavailability})}$$

when bioavailability is the characteristic attributable to the toxicant that defines its ability to be assimilated by the organism. Since it can be argued that hazard is an inverse function of safety, it may be simply stated that:

$$\text{Hazard} \propto (\text{Toxicity} \times \text{Bioavailability})$$

provided that it is accepted that hazard here refers to toxic hazard only (i.e. other hazards, such as explosivity, are disregarded).

Thresholds to the occurrence of acute effects are difficult to quantify but can be important (Hermann, 1971; Farmer, 1974; Haley *et al.*, 1974, 1975a, and 1975b). In his so-called *'Non-concept'* of *'No-threshold'* Dinman (1972) warned that to believe that a single molecule's presence in a cell implies a definitive potential for deleterious effect disregards stochastic considerations.

The hypothesis that every individual carries from birth a genetically endowed term of life beyond which it is impossible to survive is both biologically and mathematically attractive (Clarke, 1950). Acute toxicology is concerned with the influence of molecules entering the organisms and altering this term, generally in an adverse sense, and this is compatible with the physical concept of entropy change (i.e. the measure of the time progression of a bio-group from organization to disorganization).

THE OBJECTIVES OF ACUTE TOXICITY TESTS

In the experimental toxicology of pesticides to vertebrates the objectives of acute toxicity tests are:

(i) To predict hazard to non-target species.
(ii) To assess toxicity in target species when the pest is a vertebrate animal.
(iii) To provide information on the mechanism of toxic action.
(iv) To provide data on which user risk–benefit relationships may be assessed.
(v) To aid the establishment of exposure levels in studies designed to assess long-term effects in experimental toxicology.

These objectives together with the experimental variants, route of exposure, test animals, dose, and response form the main subject of this book.

Undoubtedly the most commonly used experimental procedure for assessing and quantifying acute toxicity is the so-called 'LD_{50} test' (Chapter 2). However, the late Lord Platt, a former President of the Royal College of Physicians and from 1961 to 1972 a member of the U.K. Home Office Advisory Committee on the Cruelty to Animals Act, 1876 is attributed as stating to the House of Lords: 'The LD_{50} is most extravagant in the use of animals; it is questionable whether it is morally or ethically sound in most cases and whether it gives the results we want to answer the questions we need to put'. A corollary to this and other criticism of the 'LD_{50} test' has been the initiation in the U.K. in 1977 of an investigative panel charged with reporting to the U.K. Home Office Advisory Committee on the Cruelty to Animals Act, 1876. The panel had expert assessors and the following terms of reference:

> To enquire into the experimental procedure involving living animals which is known as the LD_{50} test and to taken such written and oral evidence for this purpose as may seem appropriate; to consider:
>
> (a) the extent of its use in accordance with statutory requirements and otherwise, and
> (b) the scientific necessity and justification for the test in its various applications;
>
> and to make any recommendations to the Secretary of State they may consider appropriate about the exercise of his powers under the Cruelty to Animals Act, 1876, in relation to this test.

The findings of the Panel were reported by the Home Office in 1979.[a]

It is the opinion of many toxicologists that there is a need for detailed information on the acute toxicity of all pesticides and pesticide formulations in order that judgements can be made on safety and hazard. However, this does not imply that toxicologists are satisfied that adequate attention is being given to the design, performance, and interpretations of many of the acute toxicity tests currently required nor does it suggest that toxicologists would not welcome procedures that do not involve the use of living animals. Unfortunately, in the current state of knowledge there is little hope that the use of sentient species for investigative acute toxicity tests will be replaced by techniques such as tissue and organ culture (Desi *et al.*, 1977) or the use of bird embryos (Marliac *et al.*, 1965). The use of computerized structure–toxicity analysis (Enslein *et al.*, 1977) and computerized data banking, as is being initiated by the U.S. Environmental Protection Agency, will slightly decrease the number of tests performed but it will be a long time before a significant diminution is observed.

[a]*Report on the LD_{50} Test*—Presented to the Secretary of State by the Advisory Committee on the Administration of the Cruelty to Animals Act 1876. Home Office, London, 1979.

CHAPTER 1

Prologue—justification of the need for acute toxicity information for pesticides

It has been estimated that out of the present world population of 3.9×10^9 people (U.N. Statistical Office estimate of world population at mid-1975) some 500×10^6 suffer malnutrition and more than $1\,500 \times 10^6$ are underfed. The situation can be expected to worsen since the estimated world population will rise to between 5.4 and 6.9×10^9 by the year 2000 (U.N. forecasts quoted by Ehrlich and Ehrlich, 1970). By carrying out calculations in average money terms, the Groupement International des Associations Nationales de Fabricants de Pesticides (GIFAP) has estimated that the loss of the world's potential harvest due to insect pests, plant diseases, and weeds, is equal to the cost of the whole of the world's grain harvest plus the cost of the world's potato harvest, or in other words, more than one-third of the potential world harvest is destroyed by pests of various types. Although there is a body of contra-opinion, the author subscribes to the view that pesticides are an integral part of modern technology and that it is doubtful that civilization could continue in its present form without the use of pesticides.[a] The major European pesticides' manufacturers have produced a book that sets out the case for and against the need for pesticides.[b]

Consistent with the above facts but illustrating something of the complexity of economic arguments for and against the use of pesticides are the two examples that follow. It has been estimated by the Environmental Protection Agency (EPA) in the U.S.A. that the ban on the use of six pesticides (DDT, chlordane, heptachlor, aldrin, dieldrin, and organomercurials) will cost U.S. residents only the equivalent of 5 cents each per year, based on predictions for the period 1973 to 1985.[c] The Philippines, a fiscally poor country, currently loses 50×10^6 (U.S.A.) dollars worth of its essential rice crop every year owing to infestation by

[a]'Pesticides in the Modern World'—A symposium prepared by members of the Co-operative Programme of Agro-Allied Industries with FAO and other United Nations Organizations (1972).
[b]*Pesticides and Human Welfare*, Editors: D. L. Gunn and J. G. R. Stevens (Oxford University Press, 1976).
[c]Environmental Protection Agency (U.S.A.) estimates quoted in *Pesticide and Toxic Chemicals News*, **5**, 12 (1977).

rats despite the multiplicity of rodenticides available.[d] Based on this type of observation it must be accepted that not all the pesticides that are used are essential and also that many good pesticides are not used in the most effective manner.

Considering the acutely toxic nature of many pesticides and the vast amounts manufactured and distributed (Waitt, 1975); in 1974 over 9 × 10^8 lb of pesticides were used by agricultural, governmental, and industrial users in the U.S.A. alone, thus it is remarkable that there are so few fatalities or other overt intoxications. For example, there are approximately 100 organophosphorus pesticides currently in use and these account for an annual world-wide production exceeding 2 × 10^8 lb (Casida and Baron 1976) and some of these products are highly toxic to non-target species.[e] Authenticated data on pesticide intoxications are hard to obtain since many of the major users are in the less developed areas of the world where even elementary levels of protection are not used (e.g. the employment of illiterate peasants or even children as pesticide applicators is not uncommon in some countries) and adequate medical or other incident records are not kept. It must be recalled that many highly toxic pesticides can be handled safely provided that the operators are dressed in the correct protective equipment and observe reasonable precautions.[f] Kaloyanova-Simeonova and Fournier (1971) attempted to review the actual situation with regard to pesticide intoxications in man and the World Health Organization has produced various reports on the subject.[g,h] According to World Health Organization estimates published in 1973,[i] there are about 500 × 10^3 cases of acute accidental pesticide poisoning in the world each year and between 1 and 10% of these are fatal.

The geographical and/or ethnic distribution of the statistics quoted by the World Health Organization are not fully documented in the published literature. It is pertinent to consider the documented facts for the United Kingdom and the U.S.A., both countries having developed data banks on this subject. Hearn (1973) reviewed in detail all pesticide incidents that were reported in England and Wales during the period 1952–1971; during that period there were only 9 fatal cases and of those only 3 were occupational in origin. Hearn (1973) records however that there were

[d]Editorial, *Rice Journal*, **79**, 6–7 (1976).
[e]'Recommended Classification of Pesticides by Hazard' *Wld. Hlth. Org. Chronicle*, **29**, 397–401 (1975).
[f]*Proceedings of the National Conference on Protective Clothing and Safety Equipment for Pesticide Workers*. (Federal Working Group on Pest Management), Rockville, Md., U.S.A. (1972).
[g]*Modern Trends in the Prevention of Pesticide Intoxications*. Wld. Hlth. Org. Report on the conference held at Kiev, U.S.S.R. 1971. (Published by Wld. Hlth. Org. Regional Bureau for Europe, Copenhagen, Denmark.)
[h]'Epidemiological Toxicology of Pesticide Exposure—Report of an International Workshop.' *Arch. Environ. Hlth.*, **25**, 339–405 (1972).
[i]Wld. Hlth. Org. 25th Anniversary Series on major public health problems.

actually 121 cases of systemic intoxication, including the 9 fatalities. To put these figures into some perspective it is necessary to consider the data from the Chief Safety Inspector of the U.K. Ministry of Agriculture, Fisheries, and Food.[j] For the four year period 1968–1971, there were a total of 157 deaths caused by tractors and 65 deaths due to falls by agricultural and horticultural workers in the United Kingdom, but during that same period there were no deaths due to acute intoxication by pesticides. Even with a safety record such as that, complacency must be avoided and Clutterbuck,[k] writing in a British trade union journal, has addressed a strong warning to agricultural workers about the threat of poisoning from pesticide sprays.

In the U.S.A. during the decade 1950–1960, there was approximately 1 per 100×10^3 deaths per annum due to intoxication by liquids and solids. According to Cann (1963), 6–10% of these deaths were due to pesticides. To put some perspective to these figures, it must be realized that during the period 1950–1968 there was a world increase in the use of pesticides that may be represented by a financial value of £200 $\times 10^6$ increased to £1 230 $\times 10^6$, that is a sixfold increase of which the North American Continent accounted for some 50% (Galley, 1973 quoted in a paper by Waitt, 1975). In the number of fatalities quoted an important toxicological bias occurs, for during that period (i.e. 1950–1960) 30% of the fatalities in the U.S.A. occurred in the population of children under the age of 5 years and the mortality rate was about 2 : 1 non-white to white children. Lisella (1972) has quoted figures for pesticide poisoning obtained from the U.S. Poisons Control Center, as follows:

Year	Number of reported poisonings	Number of fatalities
1968	5 739	24
1969	5 702	26
1970	5 729	21

The actual number of poisonings may well be in excess of these figures as there is no certainty that all cases are reported, in fact in a later survey Hayes (1977) has reported a figure of 56 deaths in 1969. Following a careful check on the death certificates issued, the U.S. National Center for Health Statistics has reported (Hayes, 1977) the following number of

[j]Data from the Chief Safety Inspector, U.K. Ministry of Agriculture, Fisheries, and Food quoted by J. M. Barnes (1973), *Outlook on Agriculture*, 7, 97–101.
[k]'Threat of poisoning from pesticide sprays exposed.' Article by Dr C. Clutterbuck of the British Society for Social Responsibility in Science in *Land Worker* (October), 1976.

deaths due to pesticides in U.S.A.:

Year	Number of fatalities
1961	100 (approx.)
1969	56
1973	32
1974	35

The comment was made that most poisonings were non-occupational and involved gross carelessness.

As a generality, Hamilton and Hardy (1974) have estimated that each year in the U.S.A. there is about one fatality per million of population caused by pesticides and there is about one non-fatal pesticide intoxication per ten thousand of population. In the U.S.A., as in any other country, outbreaks of poisoning due to a specific cause may distort the statistics, as for example, the large number of people intoxicated by one particular arsenical rodenticide in Memphis, Tennessee (Lovejoy, 1975), where there were 34 recorded cases of arsenical poisoning during the period between 1971 and 1973, this despite the well-known acute toxicity of arsenical pesticides in laboratory animals and man (Done and Peart, 1971). Even with these statistical aberrations, Davies (1972) has correlated the ethnic distribution of pesticide accidents in the U.S.A. with the demographic profile of the agricultural working population.

Apart from the actual poisoning of people handling agricultural chemicals, accidents will continue to occur. For example, there has been a recent incident report of 3 people killed and 300 hospitalized in the Philippines owing to thiodan contaminated flour being made into bread.[l] Factory explosions and fires may release toxicants, as happened at Seveso, Italy, when chlorophenols (commonly used as intermediates in the manufacture of agricultural chemicals) were pyrolysed to form the more toxic 2,3,7,8-tetrachlorodibenzo-p-dioxin and this, as well as chlorophenols was spread over a wide area around the factory (Reggiani, 1978); a comparable, but fortunately more contained, incident has previously occurred at another factory in Derbyshire, England (May, 1973). Acute oral LD_{50} values of 0.022 mg/kg for male rats and 0.045 mg/kg for female rats and an even lower value of 0.000 6 mg/kg for the LD_{50} value in guinea-pigs have been reported.[m]

Because of the poor standards of industrial hygiene, leptophos, a

[l]Report in the *Daily Telegraph* dated 14 February 1977.
[m]"Report on 2,4,5-T'—A report of the panel on herbicides of the President's Science Advisory Committee (Executive Office of the President of the U.S.A.—March, 1971).

neurotoxic organophosphorus insecticide, has caused severe adverse effects in operatives in a manufacturing plant in the U.S.A., whereas the same pesticide has been manufactured without adverse effects in Japan, thus demonstrating that even noxious chemicals can be handled safely if adequate precautions are imposed.

The herbicide paraquat has been the cause of numerous deaths throughout the world. Most, if not all, of the deaths have been attributable to misuse of the product (i.e. murder, suicide or accidental ingestion from unlabelled and unsuitable containers); Staiff et al. (1975) and Van Dijk et al. (1975) are among the many who have published on this subject. It is perhaps surprising that out of the vast knowledge of paraquat intoxication in animals and man, so far, no effective antidote has been discovered (Rose, 1975; Goulding et al., 1976) although some advances have been made (Fairshter and Wilson, 1975; Cavelli and Fletcher, 1977). The otherwise excellent safety record of paraquat in use is attributable to the influence of formulation, hence the commonly used granules of paraquat are only classified as Class III (slightly hazardous) and the 20% liquid formulation as Class II (moderately hazardous) in the World Health Organization Classification of Pesticides by Hazard.[e]

Theobald Smith, addressing the Philadelphia Pathological Society in 1900, enunciated the principle that man frequently attempts the conquest of problems from the least accessible quarter.[n] This principle may be believed by some to be true of the acute toxicity tests applied to pesticides, certainly Goulding (1969), addressing the British Insecticide and Fungicide Conference, expressed some criticism of the approach of toxicologists and legislators to the subject. One way in which attempts have been made to rationalize the study of acute toxicity has been the attempted correlation of chemical and physical properties with the acute toxicity data obtained from each chemical. The use by Ferguson (1939) of chemical potential as an indicator, the use of substituents on known molecules (as exemplified by Schrader (1961) with organophosphorus insecticides), and the analysis of physico-chemical variables by Free and Wilson (1964). Hudson et al. (1970), Hansch (1970), Craig (1973), have all led to the suggestion that the acute toxicities of compounds can be predicted by the use of a computer. The Environmental Protection Agency of the U.S.A. is undertaking the formation of a computer base with the objective of predicting LD_{50} values.[o] Enslein et al. (1977) have developed a statistical method based on three parameters only: chemical structure, partition coefficient, and molecular weight, but the total validity of this approach has still to be established.

Gold (1977) has explained that in the formulation of an equation to

[n]Theobald Smith quoted by Leader, R. W. (1969). Fed. Proc., **28**, 1804–1809.
[o]Environmental Protection Agency (U.S.A.) quoted in Pestic. Tox. Chem. News, **5**, 4–6 (1977).

describe a dynamic process, one begins by constructing a mental image of the elementary events that comprise the overall process and that the construction of such a mental image is based on accumulated biological and physical knowledge of the system; depending heavily on the 'biological intuition' of the modeller. Gold's description of events is very pertinent to the idea of modelling in predictive acute toxicology.

One reason for scepticism about the inanimate approach to predicting acute toxicity is that many closely related chemicals are toxic because of quite different modes of action. For example, the two chemically related herbicides diquat (1,1'-ethylene-2,2'-bipyridilium) and paraquat (1,1'-dimethyl-4,4'-bipyridilium) are toxic to mammals via entirely different targets, paraquat primarily attacking the lungs (Murray and Gibson, 1972 and 1974) whereas diquat causes a massive shift of fluid from the tissues into the lumen of the gastro-intestinal tract (Crabtree et al., 1977; Crabtree and Rose, 1978).

In the present state of knowledge interspecies variation in sensitivity to toxicants cannot sensibly be predicted by the use of computers although there must also be some misgivings about predictive animal tests involving extrapolation from one species to another. The rodenticide N-3-pyridylmethyl-N'-p-nitrophenyl urea has been demonstrated as requiring 200 times the rat lethal dose to kill monkeys, but in South Korea there have been at least seven fatalities attributable to the use of this rodenticide,[p] thus suggesting that even the use of primates may not be a better indicator of human risk than some of the lower vertebrates. Observations of this type inevitably raise questions as to the rationale of choice of laboratory animals for acute toxicity testing with pesticides (see Chapter 3).

It has been stated that the toxicity of a product is its capacity to cause injury while the hazard attributable to the product represents the probability that it will do so (Barnes, 1963). Quite clearly it is possible to invest a lot of effort in producing statistically attractive data on effects and doses and still miss the obvious enormous variability due to species differences and ambient conditions. Weil (1972a), in a definitive paper on statistics and safety factors, indicated clearly the folly of attempting to use data generated for the assessment of LD_{50} values to calculate LD_y data when the value of y is less than 50%, indeed even values of y as close to the mid-point as 35% were shown by Weil to be very inaccurate. However, on the basis of a statement published by Hayes (1971) on the importance of low-level exposure of pesticide workers to anticholinesterase agents, Haley et al. (1974a and 1974b, 1975a, and 1975b) have determined acute toxicity values for several carbamates, organophosphates, and organothiophosphates down to the $LD_{0.1}$ values and lower. It is interesting

[p]'Rodenticide blamed for Korean deaths' reported in *Chemical and Engineering News*, 7 July 1975.

that Hayes's (1971) suggestion that anticholinesterase pesticides may be the cause of sub-lethal effects in agricultural workers has been more recently confirmed in the U.S.A. by Quinones *et al*. (1976) and again there was an ethnic factor involved as all the cases studied were migrant farm workers of Puerto Rican ancestry and all the pesticides used (parathion, methylparathion, malathion, and carbaryl) had been intensively studied over many years. Attempts have been made to set standards for monitoring exposure to anticholinesterase agents (Long, 1975; Gervais, 1976) and an experimental protocol for the field assessment of exposure by spraymen and others has been distributed through the offices of the World Health Organization (Division of Vector Biology and Control).

The exposure of operators to pesticides can sometimes be monitored by analysis of concentrations in the blood (e.g. dieldrin exposure can be measured by the method of Brown *et al*., 1964) or the determination of excreted pesticide or metabolites in the urine (Cueto and Biros, 1967). The interpretation of these types of data requires care in relation to the acute toxicity situation and cognizance must be taken of the principles of pharmacokinetics involved.

The World Health Organization has published monographs on the subject of monitoring humans for pesticide exposure,[q,r] and in the U.S.A., a Federal Working Group on Pest Management[s] set out guidelines for monitoring human exposure to pesticides.

Even with well controlled agricultural and horticultural practices in the United Kingdom adventitious exposures do occur. An examination of the national and local newspapers can reveal this type of incident, as for example three fairly important incidents all within a few days in one month of 1977 in England. In Lincolnshire 50 children in a school playground were affected by pesticide spray drift, fortunately none of the children was seriously intoxicated.[t] In Kent, a farm worker had to be admitted to hospital after inhaling pesticide being sprayed from a helicopter.[u] In Cambridgeshire, firemen, policemen, and ambulancemen were all affected by pesticide when dealing with a crashed crop-spraying aircraft.[v] Although seasonal, this number of incidents was not unusual. The potential for disastrous acute intoxications in other less technically and less socially advanced countries must be proportionately greater.

Fournier (1974), writing on the toxicity of pesticides to humans, stated that acute exposures occur as a result of voluntary absorption more often than as a result of occupational handling of products. This being the case,

[q]'Safe Use of Pesticides' (20th Report of WHO Expert Committee on Insecticides).
[r]'Chemical and Biochemical Methodology for the Assessment of Hazard of Pesticides for Man', Wld. Hlth. Org. Techn. Rep. Ser. 1975, No. 560.
[s]Guidelines by U.S.A. Federal Working Group on Pest Management (1974) outlined in paper by Long, K. R. (1975). *Int. Arch. Occup. Environ. Hlth.*, **36**, 75–86.
[t]Report in *The Times* dated 15 July 1977.
[u]Report in *The Kent Messenger* dated 22 July 1977.
[v]Report in *The Times* dated 29 July 1977.

some pesticides that are very toxic by ingestion are capable of being handled safely because of poor skin penetrating properties. This combination of characteristics is frequently found with the carbamate insecticides, for example carbofuran has an acute oral LD_{50} value of about 11 mg/kg in the rat, but has an acute percutaneous toxicity of 10.2 g/kg in the same species (Tobin, 1970). Certainly Fournier's statement has been true in relation to the number of human intoxications that have occurred with the quaternary herbicides.

Carbofuran

In addition to concern for acute pesticide intoxications involving humans, the toxicologist must also be aware of the potential for acute intoxications by pesticides in sub-human non-target species. These may include domesticated, economic and pet animals (Clarke and Clarke, 1975) and wild animals (De Witt, 1966). In the wild, sub-lethal acute intoxication can easily lead to fatalities due to secondary effects (e.g. predation); thus LD_{50} value may be of very limited interest under these conditions.

What follows in this monograph is an examination of the importance and meaning of acute tests in the toxicology of pesticides to vertebrates in the hope that a critical review of the subject may lead to advances in the techniques of predictive acute toxicity testing and reveal ways in which the results of such tests may be used more meaningfully in the development and safe use of pesticides.

CHAPTER 2

Responses

Acute exposure to pesticides may produce toxic responses that are either sub-lethal or lethal. For example, the anthelmintic haloxon can cause delayed neurotoxicity in some, but not all, species (Malone, 1964) and the insecticide mipafox has caused paralysis in man (Bidstrup *et al.*, 1953); the soil fumigant methyl bromide has caused neurological disorders in man (Jordi, 1953; Collins, 1965). At sub-cellular level, some organophosphates have been demonstrated as causing chromosome damage (Trinh-Van-Bao *et al.*, 1974) and even psychiatric disorders have been known to follow acute pesticide exposures (Conyers and Goldsmith, 1971).

The signs and symptoms of acute intoxications may be overt or subtle (Medved *et al.*, 1964; Namba, 1971; Jovic, 1974; Silverman, 1974). Sometimes the overt signs may mask the subtle signs but it may be possible and meaningful to isolate the subtle toxic responses and to quantify them (Aston *et al.*, 1962; Vandekar *et al.*, 1965; Haley *et al.*, 1974). This unmasking of the subtle effects is more commonly undertaken with therapeutic agents than with pesticides (Meeter *et al.*, 1971). Revzin (1973a, 1973b, 1976a and 1976b) reported that anticholinesterase insecticides can affect attention and short-term memory through effects on the hippocampus at doses too low to induce detectable peripheral symptomatology, and also the use of atropine to overcome anticholinesterase intoxication may actually synergize these subtle effects; interestingly, Revzin found that the pigeon was a good model for this research and as a consequence recommended extreme caution in the handling of anticholinesterase agents by aerial applicators.

Cerebral oedema is a subtle toxic effect that can occur following exposure to some organotin compounds (Kimbrough, 1976) and is an example of a potential subtle hazard that must be investigated in relation to the acute toxicity of organotin pesticides.

Since it is not possible to obtain information on symptoms, as distinct from signs of intoxication, from experimental animals valuable toxicological information may be inaccessible. Because of the subjective nature of symptoms, even information on these from humans may be inaccurate and suspect. Because of the incomplete information available all extrapolations of information from one species to another and interpretations of observations must be carried out cautiously (Perlman, 1970) and, in addition to the obvious overt signs of intoxication, physical and behavioural changes should be assessed (Aston *et al.*, 1962; Levin, 1974;

14

Rodnitzky, 1974; Reiter *et al.*, 1973 and 1975). In relation to pesticides, most behavioural studies have been carried out with cholinesterase inhibitors (Russell *et al.*, 1961; Goldberg *et al.*, 1963; Glow and Rose, 1965; Durham *et al.*, 1965; Reiter *et al.*, 1973 and 1975; Bignami *et al.*, 1975; Levin and Rodnitzky, 1976) and with organochlorine insecticides (Van Gelder, 1975).

The qualitative response to toxicants under conditions of acute exposure has been classified into four types by McLean (1971):

(i) Non-specific

Essentially the non-specific response is a mass-action effect and, since pesticides are by definition biocidal, this type of response is rare in pesticide toxicology. The acute toxicity of piperonyl butoxide (Brown 1970) may be considered to be an illustrative example of this mechanism although piperonyl butoxide is strictly not a pesticide but is used to synergize some other chemicals with pesticidal properties.

(ii) Reactive

Reactive toxicants are capable of attacking diverse chemical groups in cells and by this means they destroy the function of the cells. For example, the quaternary herbicide paraquat (Clark, *et al.*, 1966; Kimbrough and Gaines, 1970) with its selective reactive effects on lung tissues and another related herbicide, morfamquat, with its specific toxic effects on the proximal convoluted tubules of kidneys (Calderbank, 1968; Balogh and Merk, 1973), are both examples of the reactive class of toxicants. However, diquat, a close chemical relation to paraquat and morfamquat does not have this reactivity (Oreopoulos and McEvoy, 1969; Clark and Hurst, 1970), this is due, at least in part, to the overall distribution and excretion

Paraquat

Diquat

Morfamquat

pattern differences of the three quaternary herbicides (Daniel and Gage, 1966; Litchfield *et al.*, 1973).

(iii) Highly specific

With all pesticides that are toxic because of a direct action causing inhibition of enzymes, such as most pesticidal carbamates and some organophosphates, the toxic response may manifest itself in a more complex syndrome (Meeter and Wolthuis, 1968) but the origin of the response is highly specific. The highly specific response may require very defined characteristics in the pesticide molecule, for example optical isomers may behave differently (Spencer, 1961; Morello *et al.*, 1967 and 1968) or in the receptor species (Donninger, 1971).

(iv) Those requiring modification before becoming fully toxic

The term 'lethal synthesis' was coined to describe this type of metabolic modification (Peters, 1963). There are several examples of pesticides that are not particularly active as the parent compound but become toxic because of metabolism. Sodium fluoroacetate is used as a rodenticide because it is converted *in vivo* to the fluorocitrate and this is a highly toxic product, not only to rodents, but to many other vertebrate animals (Peters, 1963; Buffa *et al.*, 1973). Some sulphur-containing pesticides are converted *in vivo* into their more toxic oxygen analogues, for example, parathion is metabolized to paraoxon (Holtz and Westerman, 1959; Gaines *et al.*, 1966).

$$O_2N-\!\!\left\langle\!\!\underset{}{\bigcirc}\!\!\right\rangle\!\!-O-\underset{\underset{OEt}{|}}{\overset{\overset{X}{|}}{P}}-OEt \qquad \begin{array}{l} X = S,\ parathion \\ X = O,\ paraoxon \end{array}$$

Because toxic responses are frequently complexes of several interactions, more than one of McLean's definitive types may be applicable to a toxicant. The nitrophenols and halophenols, for example, cause the uncoupling of oxidative phosphorylation and hence, at lethal exposure levels, death due to respiratory failure and hypothermia, the *post-mortem* effect being characterized by rapid rigor. The toxicity of these nitro- or halophenols could be classified as reactive or as highly specific depending on the interpretation of the process of oxidative phosphorylation (Straub, 1974).

Although not included in McLean's definitions, some toxicants can cause physiological changes and these allow redistribution of the toxicant to susceptible sites in the body, thus there is a 'lethal redistribution'. The thallium salts used as rodenticides are examples of this phenomenon. Weinig and Walz (1971) demonstrated a redistribution of thallium in the kidneys and livers of rats before death. Sometimes 'lethal redistribution' is associated quite simply with the change in body weight before death (Sharp *et al*., 1972). Hayes (1974) investigated the distribution of dieldrin in the bodies of rats following exposure to a single oral dose and he concluded that a postulated model for the distribution of the insecticide in the various tissues based on the known pharmacokinetics of thiopental was incorrect; this is indicative of the danger of applying a mathematical model to a new situation without adequate supporting data from experiments.

While defining criteria for the evaluation of chemical toxicity, Princi (1964) stated that agents do not create new functions in a cell or tissue but they only modify existing functions, or at most make evident functions that were previously latent. Goldwater (1968) observed that toxicologic phenomena cannot always be predicted with accuracy or explained on the basis of physical or chemical laws and that it is this unpredictability that frequently reduces conclusions and decisions in toxicology to opinion rather than fact.

To aid interpretation in this inexact investigative process statistical inferences are commonly used. Fundamental to almost all the biometrics of acute toxicology is the relationship of the biological response to the log-normal distribution (Koch, 1966 and 1969), and commonly acute toxicity is assessed and expressed in terms of statistical principles based on population effects (Deichman and Mergard, 1948; Bliss, 1957; Bein, 1963; Hodge, 1965; Brown, 1966; Finney, 1971; Weil, 1972a and 1972b). Much of this type of approach to the subject is based on the true quantal response, however in acute toxicity studies the use of the polychotomous quantal response is quite feasible. In the true quantal response situation there are only two possible outcomes (i.e. 'All' or 'None'), whereas in the polychotomous quantal response three or more outcomes are acceptable, thus:

Alive or dead outcome = quantal response

but,   Alive—moribund—dead = polychotomous quantal response

and methods for the quantification of these latter types of data have been described by Bross (1958), Ashford (1959), and by Gurland *et al*. (1960).

Most often acute toxic effects are expressed as per cent incidence occurring in an exposed population. The symbols ED are conventionally used to indicate 'Effect Dose' and when the effect is specifically death the symbol used is LD (i.e. 'Lethal Dose'). The percentage effect is expressed as a subscript, thus if the effect were produced in 10% of the exposed population this would be written as the ED_{10}, similarly if 50% of the exposed population were killed as a result of the exposure, this would be written as LD_{50}. Sometimes the 50% effective dose or 50% lethal dose is written as MED (Median Effect Dose) or MLD (Median Lethal Dose). An alternative nomenclature is based on survival as an effect and the 'Threshold Limit' (TL) for percentage survival is written with the percentage figure as a subscript, for example TL_{50}, this must not be confused with the alternative threshold limit which is the maximum dose at which mortality does not occur.

Because of its relative precision when compared with the assessment of other dose-responses, the 50% incidence of effect is most commonly used as the expression of acute toxicity of a product (Hodge, 1965; Wilks, 1971). The great importance of much smaller percentage values in assessing the toxicity of pesticides has been demonstrated with some methylcarbamates, organophosphates, and organothiophosphates by Haley et al. (1974, 1975a, and 1975b). By using the log–normal relationship applicable to quantal responses, it is possible to calculate the theoretical threshold for any toxic manifestation that is being measured (Hermann, 1967; Haley et al., 1974a and b, 1975a, and 1975b; Farmer, 1974). Weil (1972a and 1972b) showed experimentally that there could be a wide disparity between the calculated (i.e. theoretical) and real (i.e. actually obtained) values for lethal doses even as close to the mid-point as the LD_{35} values for products. The use of log-log plots and even Arrhenius plots (i.e. log-rate plotted against the reciprocal of absolute temperature) has been shown to produce linear relationships for many biological data in relatively simple systems. Borgmann (1974) expanded the theoretical applications of this finding to more complex biological happenings and it is probable that this linear relationship will have ramifications into acute toxicity phenomena. The sort of area in which Borgmann's ideas might have application can be exemplified by the work of Cornwell and Bull (1967) and Cornwell (1969); these investigators of the acute toxicity of alphachloralose to mice found that large mice were relatively insensitive to intoxication when compared with small mice at an ambient temperature of about 18 °C but if the ambient temperature was dropped to about 13 °C, the sensitivity differential disappeared and there was an overall increase in the susceptibility of the mice to intoxication.

In order to assess the ED_y when y is some required happening expressed as a percentage, it is not necessary to actually achieve the event at the defined level. All that is required is a sufficient number of estimates of y between 0 and 100% in order to apply the mathematical principles that have been derived from the study of biological response curves (Westerfeld, 1956; Koch, 1966 and 1969). The earliest statistical analysis to be commonly used for this purpose was that of Kärber (1931) but his method was severely criticized by Thompson (1947), and Kärber's approach to the problem was subjected to a detailed critique by Bross (1950). Because of the interest in lethality of chemicals to microbial populations, a lot of impetus to improving the precision of effective dose estimates occurred in relation to bacteriology and related subjects (Wilson and Worcester, 1943a and 1943b; Worcester and Wilson, 1943; Thompson, 1947). Following this, Weil et al. (1953) reported on their experiences with the statistical analysis of acute toxicity data. Out of these independent investigations and adaptions of Thompson's (1947) method involving moving averages and the interpolation of data to estimate the median effective dose was rationalized to tabular form by Thompson and Weil (1952) and further developed by Weil (1952). These so-called 'Moving Average' methods are still commonly used in toxicology.

Bliss (1935a, 1935b, and 1938) who was working in biological assay provided the basis for a whole branch of biometrics called Probit Analysis, and this was further developed mathematically by Finney (1971). Miller and Tainter (1944) described a convenient method by which ED_{50} values could be calculated by simply plotting the log-dose against the Probit of the response on suitable graph paper. In a quantal situation, if a graph is plotted of response on a linear scale against either the dose on a linear scale or the log-dose then sigmoid curves will result (Westerfeld, 1956). This is illustrated in Figures 2.1 and 2.2 using data for the acute oral toxicity of an aqueous solution of tetramethylammonium chloride to rats, but since the response data can be considered to be random, the principle of maximum likelihood holds good and the sigmoid curve is applicable when x is the dose used.

If μ (Figure 2.2) is taken to be the value of x corresponding to the dose

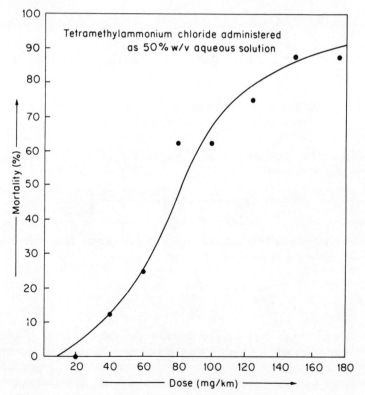

Figure 2.1 The acute oral toxicity of tetramethylammonium chloride to adult (CFE strain) rats displayed on a linear scale

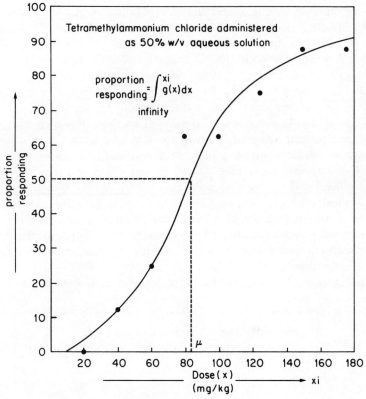

Figure 2.2 The acute oral toxicity of tetramethylammonium chloride to adult (CFE strain) rats displayed on a linear scale

producing a 50% response (i.e. the LD_{50} or the ED_{50}), then the following equation can be derived:

$$g(x) = \frac{I}{\sqrt{2\pi\sigma}} \exp\left(-\frac{(x - \mu)^2}{2\sigma^2}\right)$$

However, Gaddum (1933) showed that if the response data were modified by the arbitrary use of the value 5 in the equation:

$$P = \frac{I}{\sqrt{2\pi}} \int_{-\infty}^{t-5} e^{-x^2/2} dx$$

and the term 'Probit' was used to describe the value P (N.B. 'Probit' was derived from 'Probability Unit'), then if this is substituted on the ordinate in Figure 2.1 and the dose shown in the abscissa is converted to a log-scale, the sigmoid curve is transformed to a straight-line form, as shown in Figure 2.3.

There have been numerous detailed accounts of the use of Probit

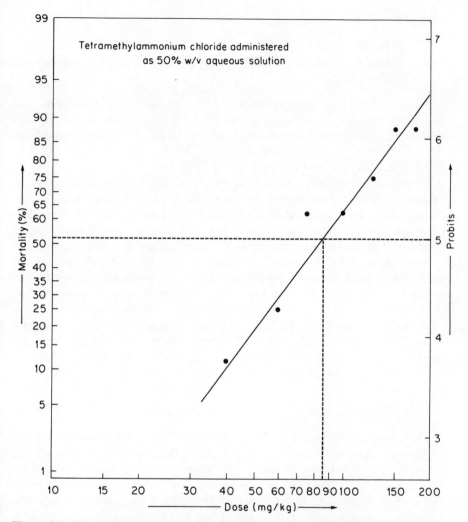

Figure 2.3 The acute oral toxicity of tetramethylammonium chloride to adult (CFE strain) rats displayed on a Probit-Log dose scale

Analysis in bioassay (e.g. Cornfield, 1964; Miller, 1964; Dews and Berkson, 1964; Bliss, 1964; Dunnett, 1968) but the fullest account of the process is attributable to Finney (1971). Knudsen and Curtis (1947) described the use of angular transformation in the analysis of bioassay data and Waud (1972) has written a detailed mathematical analysis of this and related data transformations in the quantal process.

In another publication Waud (1975) suggested the use of the logistic function:

$$P = \frac{D^E}{(D^E + K^E)}$$

where, P = probability of response

D = dose

E and K are scale and location parameters in which K corresponds to the ED_{50}.

Waud (1972) earlier demonstrated by an iterative technique that maximum likelihood equations can be set up for estimating K and E, such that the value for the ED_{50} can be expected to lie within some confidence band. The use of the logistic function for this purpose was not new (Berkson, 1944) but had not been widely adopted.

In the more complex situation in which polychotomous data are to be calculated Ridit Analysis may be used (Bross, 1958). The 'Ridit' (N.B. 'Ridit' was derived from the expression 'Relative to an identified distribution') is relative to an empirical distribution and differs from a Probit in that the latter is relative to a theoretical distribution.

Some finite time limits are generally set for the exposure or for the response or both in acute toxicology. There are mathematical techniques for dealing quantitatively with the time limitation in an assessment (Bishop *et al.*, 1971), but in practice these techniques are seldom applied.

Although graphical methods are available (Miller and Tainter, 1944; De Beer, 1945; Litchfield and Wilcoxon, 1949) and tables for easy computation are published (Thompson and Weil, 1952; Weil, 1952) it is very convenient to utilize modern computer techniques for the rapid calculation of acute data via Probit Analysis (Fink and Hund, 1965; Spratt, 1966; Daum and Killcreas, 1966; Davies, 1971) or other stochastic methods (Cochran and Davis, 1964).

The assessment of acute toxicity in terms of ED_y or LD_y values when y is a specified percentage must be imprecise as the populations used are not infinitely large and, in practice, are generally fairly small. Probability statistics can be applied to the estimates at any point on the dose-response line and it is usual to calculate the Confidence Limits for each point as being ± 1.96 standard errors, that is the Confidence Limits at the 95% Level of Probability. Although the use of fiducial logic often gives rise to the same numerical limits as those derived by applying the principle of ± 1.96 standard errors, the term Fiducial Limits should not be used as being synonymous with Confidence Limits unless fiducial logic has been applied to the estimates although the numerical results may be the same.

Litchfield and Wilcoxon (1949) described in detail a method for estimating the Confidence Limits for the ED_{50} when the log dose–Probit method of estimation is used, the essential details, without proof, are as follows:

Estimate ED_{16} (corresponding to Probit 4) and ED_{84} (corresponding to Probit 6)

$$\text{Slope function } S = \left(\frac{ED_{84}}{ED_{50}} + \frac{ED_{50}}{ED_{16}} \right) \times \tfrac{1}{2}$$

N = Number of animals tested at those doses whose expected effects were between 16 and 84%

$$S^{\text{exponent}} = S^{2.77/N} = f\,ED_{50}$$

95% Confidence Limits for ED_{50} will be given by:

$$ED_{50} \times f\,ED_{50} = \text{Upper limit}$$

$$ED_{50} \big/ f\,ED_{50} = \text{Lower limit}$$

As an alternative to the LD_{50} values for the classification for toxic chemicals, Luckey and Venugopal (1977) have suggested that the term:

$$pT = -\text{Log}\,(T)$$

when,

T = Molar concentration of toxicant that will kill 50% of the experimental population (i.e. expressed as mol/kg bodyweight)

should be used. The advantage claimed by Luckey and Venugopal is that the numerical rating will be more readily understood by lay-people. Using this type of nomenclature it can be seen that:

if, $pT = 1$ the $LD_{50} = 0.1$ mol/kg

       $pT = 2$ the $LD_{50} = 0.01$ mol/kg

       $pT = 3$ the $LD_{50} = 0.001$ mol/kg

if the pT value is negative then the LD_{50} value must be greater than 1 mol/kg and the toxicant can be considered as 'non-toxic'. This system is not yet widely used.

The efficient design of acute toxicity studies takes into account the optimal numbers of animals to be involved at each dose level in order to achieve the desired degree of precision. This quantity will vary between different investigations and is, in part, a function of the slope (β) of the achieved log dose–Probit regression line. By using the equation:

$$V(m) = \frac{1}{\beta^2}\left(\frac{1}{\sum_t \dfrac{nz^2}{PQ}} + \frac{(m-\bar{x})^2}{\sum_t \dfrac{nz^2}{PQ}(x-\bar{x})^2}\right)$$

$V(m)$ = Variance of the estimated log LC_{50}

    n = Number of fish per treatment level

    m = Estimated log LC_{50}

    β = Slope of probit regression line

B

z = Ordinate to the normal distribution corresponding to the probability level

P = Proportion killed on average at log-concentration x

Q = Proportion not-killed on average at x

$\bar{x}$ = Mean log-concentration

x = Log-concentration

t = Number of test levels

Jensen (1972) studied the optimum number of fish for estimating lethal concentrations (LC) of toxicants. Increasing the number of fish between 1 and 10 substantially decreased the standard error of the LC_{50}, increasing the number of fish from 10 to 20 decreased the error by 29%, increasing from 20 to 30 decreased the error by 13%, thereafter, increasing numbers of fish had only a very small influence on the standard error. This general principle can be applied to all quantal estimates of ED_{50}.

In acute toxicity tests involving whole atmosphere exposures (e.g. aquatic toxicology and inhalation toxicology), the effect levels are expressed in terms of concentrations rather than doses and the conventional nomenclature becomes EC (Effect Concentration) and LC (Lethal Concentration) rather than using dose (i.e. LC_{50} corresponds to LD_{50} with the dose being expressed as a concentration in the whole atmosphere surrounding the animal).

Majda (1976) determined the LD_{50} values with 95% Confidence Limits for 47 chemicals using 10 animals per dose level, then, using statistically randomized selection of data, Majda calculated the probable LD_{50} values with limits for the use of sub-groups of 6, 5, 4, 3, or 2 animals per dose level; from the data obtained, it was found that there were only small differences in the mean LD_{50} values although when the dose group was dropped to 2 or 3 animals the confidence interval was about doubled. The cautionary statement by Finney (1971) that 'The experimenter who can afford only 10 animals and wishes to estimate the mean toxic dose of a new poison or the mean curative dose of a new therapeutic agent, however, is asking for the impossible; discussion of whether he ought to use two groups of 5 animals or to give every animal a different dose is often vigorous but always unprofitable' must always be in the mind of the toxicologist.

Regrettably the numbers of animals used by investigators to determine acute toxicity are often influenced by regulatory requirements rather than scientific necessity although it is obvious that the two should not be different.

Selection of doses for acute toxicity studies is often done empirically on the basis of experience and prior knowledge by the investigator. There are some mathematical guidelines using censored and truncated sampling

(Bishop *et al.*, 1971) and other sequential methods (Eichhorn, 1972; Eichhorn and Zacks, 1972) but the most commonly used formal approach is the so-called 'Up-and-Down' or 'Pyramid' method for small samples (Brownlee *et al.*, 1953; Dixon, 1965; Choi, 1971). The 'Up-and-Down' method has the advantage of being economical in the number of animals used but can cause logistic problems in the programming of tests and may be wasteful of test material especially if solutions have to be prepared for dosing the animals. Because of the economy of numbers of animals used, the 'Up-and-Down' method is commonly used with species that are expensive to procure and maintain (e.g. farm animals).

Interactive toxicological effects may involve exposure to two or more toxicants either simultaneously or in sequence. As there are many different pharmacokinetic influences involved, the mathematics of interactions are very complicated (Plackett and Hewlett, 1948, 1952, and 1967; Veldstra, 1956; Landahl, 1958; Hewlett, 1960 and 1969; Hewlett and Plackett, 1961) and each example of interaction must be considered separately. Interactions and their interpretation can be of importance in relation to assessing the value of antidotes to intoxication (Natoff and Reiff, 1970; Natoff, 1973).

Certain principles and definitions are very important in relation to interactive effects in the acute toxicology of pesticides. In order to illustrate these principles the case of toxicants, referred to as A, B, and C, is presented:

(i) Additive effect

The observed effect of exposure to a mixture of A, B, C, etc. was exactly that expected for the situation in which exposure has been to an equivalent dose of A or B or C, etc. alone; then the effect is additive. Subject to the proviso that the characteristics of the dose-response lines for A, B, C, etc. do not differ significantly from each other, then a reciprocal rule can be applied to the data for the acute toxicity of mixtures of toxicants as follows:

$$\frac{a}{A \times 100} + \frac{b}{B \times 100} \cdots = \frac{1}{(LD_{50} \text{ of mixture})}$$

when, a, b, etc. are percentages of A, B, etc. in the mixture and A, B, etc. are LD_{50} values for the components. An alternative formula that may be used is:

$$\frac{100}{\dfrac{a}{A} + \dfrac{b}{B} + \dfrac{c}{C} \cdots} = LD_{50} \text{ of mixture}$$

(ii) Greater than additive effects

If the toxic effect observed for a two-component mixture of A and B is greater than the effect that would be achieved by either A or B alone at an equivalent higher dose, then the result is described as a synergistic effect. There are three special forms of synergistic effect:

(a) Potentiation

Potentiation is the case in which A and B have toxicological activities that are quite different from each other but one increases the toxic effect of the other.

(b) Synergism

Synergism differs from potentiation only in that A and B may have toxicological activities that are essentially similar to each other but one increases the toxic effect of the other.

Because of the inexactness of the definition of 'similarity' and 'difference' in relation to activity, the terms potentiation and synergism are frequently used as though they were interchangeable.

These different definitions can be illustrated by reference to the insecticide malathion. If malathion is administered together with parathion the toxicity to rats is less than additive (DuBois, 1963), both malathion and parathion are organophosphorus compounds, and both inhibit cholinesterases *in vivo* after metabolism to oxygen analogues. It must be noted however that simultaneous administration of malathion and parathion to animals pretreated with atropine and a quaternary oxime (i.e. usual antidotes for intoxication by anticholinesterase agents) can reverse this situation and marked synergism of the acute toxicity of the malathion can occur (Ramakrishna and Ramachandron, 1977).

If malathion is administered with demeton, the acute toxicity is greater than additive (DuBois, 1963) but both demeton and malathion have similar modes of action and this effect can be described as synergism. Trio-*o*-tolylphosphate does not inhibit cholinesterases but if administered with malathion the acute toxicity of the mixture is substantially greater than additive (Murphy *et al.*, 1959) and this effect can be designated as potentiation.

$$(MeO)_2\underset{\underset{S}{\|}}{P}.S.\underset{\underset{CH_2CO.Et}{|}}{CH}\ \overset{\overset{O}{\|}}{C}O.Et$$

Malathion

$$
(EtO)_2\overset{\overset{\displaystyle S}{\|}}{P}.O-\underset{}{\bigcirc}-NO_2
$$

Parathion

$$
(EtO)_2\underset{\underset{\displaystyle S}{\|}}{P}.O.CH_2.CH_2.S.Et + (EtO)_2\underset{\underset{\displaystyle O}{\|}}{P}.S.CH_2.CH_2.S.Et
$$

Demeton (mixture of 2 components)

Tri-o-tolylphosphate

(c) Coalitive effect

A coalitive effect occurs when the response to the mixture of toxicants could not have been achieved by either component alone. Coalitive acute toxic effects have rarely been observed with pesticides but are known to occur with some therapeutic agents (Loewe, 1938).

(iii) Antagonistic effect

Antagonistic effects are the converse of the effects described under (ii) above. That is the toxic effect of A and B together is less than that expected for the equivalent higher doses of either A or B alone. Antagonistic effects may be achieved by pretreatment with one compound before exposure to another, this is well documented for the protective effects of some carbamates administered before exposure to organophosphates (Gordon et al., 1978). Simultaneous administration of two toxicants may give rise to less than additive toxicity (e.g. malathion and parathion, see (ii) (b) above). Most often concern with antagonism is related to the post-exposure administration of antidotes (Natoff and Reiff, 1970).

The possible interactive effects observed for a mixture of two toxicants, such as A and B, may be investigated by plotting a common response for each component on the ordinates of a graph and then plotting the same measured response for defined mixtures on the same graph; these graphs are generally called 'Isoboles' and their design and interpretation has been described in detail by De Jongh (1961). Isoboles cannot be used for mixtures of more than two active components. Isoboles only indicate the level of synergism or antagonism that occurs at the chosen level of toxicity (e.g. LD_{50}) but, because the dose-response relationship may be different for each of the two components, the interaction may be quantitatively different at different levels of acute toxicity. The magnitude of any interactive response will also be different depending on whether A and B are administered simultaneously or sequentially.

The idea of using an index value to define toxic interactions is well known. Two similar index codes have been suggested by Clausing and Bieleke (1979) and by Wysocka-Paruszewska et al. (1979). The index values (V) used by Clausing and Bieleke (1979) are obtained by the formula:

$$V = \frac{\frac{1}{2}LD_{50}A + \frac{1}{2}LD_{50}B}{LD_{50}(A + B)}$$

however, the slope functions for the individual dose-response relationships are important and, if they are low, misleading results can be obtained. Clausing and Bieleke recommend that a better value for V is obtained if the formula used is changed to:

$$V = \frac{LD_{25}A + LD_{25}B}{LD_{50}(A + B)}$$

Wysocka-Paruszewska et al. (1979) expressed the equation for deriving the value of V as:

$$V = \frac{\text{Expected } LD_{50} \text{ value of } (A + B)}{\text{Observed } LD_{50} \text{ value of } (A + B)}$$

	Value of V	
	Clausing and Bieleke (1979)	Wysocka-Paruszewska et al. (1979)
Antagonism	<0.8	<0.7
Additive	0.8–1.5	0.7–1.3
More than additive	—	1.3–1.8
Potentiation	>1.5	>1.8

It is possible for interactive effects to be different in different species. Keplinger and Deichmann (1967) demonstrated that a mixture of the two chlorinated insecticides aldrin and chlordane exhibited an antagonistic response when administered to mice but the effect was synergistic when the two compounds were administered to rats.

Aldrin

Chlordane

In practice, comparisons of acute toxicity in different species or the comparison of the toxicity of a compound in different formulations are often based on ratios between arbitrary values, most often the LD_{50} values. More meaningful information is obtained by comparing the log dose-response Probit regression lines (Janku, 1973). The 'Toxicity Index' may be utilized, especially if comparisons are to be made with a series of related chemicals (Sun, 1950), this is quite simple:

$$\text{Toxicity index} = \frac{LD_{50} \text{ of test product} \times 100}{LD_{50} \text{ of standard product}}$$

These indices should be considered as convenient approximations.

Reproducibility of response is clearly of paramount importance in experimental acute toxicity testing. This reproducibility should be achievable within a laboratory even over a long period of time (Weil *et al.*, 1966). Apart from the obvious changes in staff and technique within a laboratory, subtle changes may occur in the population of test animals (McArthur *et al.*, 1971). In order to investigate intra-laboratory reproducibility of results, numerous collaborative studies have been undertaken but unfortunately not all are fully reported in the scientific literature (Craver *et al.*, 1950; Allmark, 1951; Swoap, 1955; Youden, 1963; Griffith, 1964; Weil and Wright, 1967; Weil, 1975).

For acute toxicology to have any meaning it is essential to define the product being tested. Sometimes results are entirely confounded by the presence of impurities or breakdown products (Pellegrini and Santi, 1972; Crossland and Shea, 1973). Murphy and Cheever (1972) found that some technical diphenphos had about 100 times the effect on liver and plasma carboxylesterases than the purified material. Some phosphorothionates being studied in alcoholic solutions by Casida and Sanderson (1963) were markedly potentiated by breakdown products. The ratio of o,p'-DDT to p,p'-DDT can influence the toxicity of technical DDT to mice (Okey and Page, 1974). No doubt there are many other examples.

Differences in the response of different species to the same toxicant are common. Sometimes these differences can be attributed to variations in toxicant–protein binding. Toxicant–protein binding may involve several different bonds or forces of attraction (i.e. covalent, coordinate, ionic, hydrogen, or hydrophobic binding) and these bondings may be considered in terms of the physico-chemical Law of Mass Action and a value can be ascribed for the association constant (k). Krasner (1973) has described the derivation of k in relation to reversible toxicant–protein interactions, Variation between species mainly affects the highly specific type of toxicant (i.e. toxicants that can be categorized in McLean's type (iii)). The difference in susceptibility of rats and mice to the anticoagulant rodenticide warfarin is an example of this type of variation. Niedner *et al.* (1974) found that the binding capacity or association constant (k) for blood proteins in the rat was 125.5 whereas in the less susceptible mouse the value of k was only 17.3. Working more directly with enzymes *in vivo*, Hutson and Hathway (1967) investigated the large difference in susceptibility of dog (LD_{50} in excess of 12 000 mg/kg) and rat (LD_{50} about 12 mg/kg) to the insecticidal organophosphate chlorfenvinphos. They found that the brain cholinesterases of the dog had approximately one-tenth of the sensitivity of the brain cholinesterases of the rat to inhibition by chlorfenvinphos; these investigators did not publish k-values for protein binding.

$$\text{(EtO)}_2\overset{\displaystyle O}{\overset{\displaystyle \|}{P}}.\text{O.C:CHCl}$$

Chlorfenvinphos

Species differences with the reactive type of toxicant (McLean's type (ii)) are also common but may be due to many different factors. For example, the fungicide hexachlorobenzene has been shown to cause liver injury and porphyria in man, rat, guinea-pig, and rabbit, but generally with rodents neurological changes are prominent and are the usual cause of death whereas according to the World Health Organization (Wld. Hlth. Org. Tech. Rept No. 555, 1974) liver injury and prophyria are the cause of death in man and no neurological involvement is apparent.

$$\text{Hexachlorobenzene (structure)}$$

Hexachlorobenzene

Paraquat, the quaternary herbicide, is also an example of a compound exhibiting species variation in acute response in the reactive class of pesticidal toxicants. Paraquat is less acutely toxic to rats than to guinea-pigs or some monkeys (e.g. *Macaca fasciularis*); the lung lesions in the rat and the monkey are like those reported for man (Moriyama *et al.*, 1972; Ueteke *et al.*, 1972; Fletcher, 1974) but the lung lesions in the guinea-pig do not show the characteristic interstial fibroses found in intoxicated rat, monkey, or man (Murray and Gibson, 1972 and 1974; Witschi and Kacew, 1974).

The carbamate insecticide dimetilan was shown to have a low acute toxicity in some laboratory rodents (i.e. oral LD_{50} 47–64 mg/kg in the rat and 60–65 mg/kg in the mouse) but was found to be highly toxic to cattle (oral LD_{50} approximately 5 mg/kg).

Dimetilan

Predictably, compounds requiring *in vivo* 'lethal synthesis' may vary in their toxicity to different species. There is, for example, a factor of about 250 times between the LD_{50} values for the rodenticide sodium fluoroacetate in dogs and monkeys (Peters, 1963). This was particularly apparent with *N*-methyl-*N*-(1-naphthyl)-fluoroacetamide, a compound lethal to mites because they metabolize it to fluoroacetate, but varying greatly in its toxicity to different mammals because of their differences in ability to metabolize it (Hashimoto *et al.*, 1968):

Species	Approximate LD_{50} (mg/kg)
Monkey	>300
Mouse	200 to 300
Rat	100
Guinea-pig ⎫ Rabbit ⎬ Dog ⎭	2 to 3

According to Atzert (1971) the direct oral acute toxicity of sodium fluoroacetate has been reported as being as small as 0.056 mg/kg (LD_{50} value) in the nutria (*Myocastor coypus*). The insecticide malathion is generally rated as being of a low order of acute toxicity,[a] its relatively non-toxic nature having been demonstrated in dogs (Hazleton and Holland, 1953; Guiti and Sadeghi, 1969), rats and mice (Hazleton and Holland, 1953). Gaines (1960) reported LD_{50} values for malathion in rats of more than 1 000 mg/kg, by mouth, and in excess of 4 000 mg/kg when applied percutaneously, but Radeleff (1970) showed that malathion is much more toxic to sheep and cattle, especially calves. Some fatalities have occurred in humans (Goldman and Teitel, 1958; Sellassie and Lester, 1971) as well as behaviour changes (Kurtz, 1977) and a sub-lethal paralytic syndrom (Healy, 1959) following acute exposures.

The subject of species differences in response to acute intoxication is discussed in more detail in Chapter 3.

[a]Recommended Classification of Pesticides by Hazard (*WHO Chronicle*, 1975, **29**, 397–401).

Test animals

CHOICE OF SPECIES—THE RATIONALE

The choice of test species for predictive toxicity testing is often affected by economic considerations, by the limitations of laboratory facilities or by the problems associated with the real target species. The theoretically optimum choice would be the species considered to be at risk from pesticide intoxication, then there would be no need to extrapolate data obtained from one species to others when the findings are being applied (Murphy *et al.*, 1968; Hathway, 1970).

Pesticides are ubiquitous and the vertebrates at risk may include the natural fauna, domesticated animals, and man. Tests for the prediction of toxic hazard to wild or domesticated animals are often carried out with reasonably closely related species in the laboratory and sometimes it is possible to work with the actual species under laboratory conditions.

During the development stages of a new pesticide and during the actual use of developed pesticides the effects on feral animals can be closely observed (Walker, 1964; Crossland and Elgar, 1974); however, unforeseen events can occur such as the killing of 1 300 water buffaloes in the Nile Delta by the organophosphorus insecticide leptophos (Hamza, 1973; Abou-Donia *et al.*, 1974; Barlow, 1977), a compound demonstrated to have a low acute toxicity in several laboratory species.

What may cause reversible signs of intoxication in laboratory animals may prove to be lethal in the wild. A transient paralysis or slowing of movement may render a wild animal vulnerable to predation or other secondry effects, such as heat dehydration (Brown, V. K. H. 1974).

By the selective use of several appropriate species it is possible to consider laboratory findings in the context of ecosystems (Howard *et al.*, 1968) but caution is essential in the design and interpretation of such models. Many toxic effects in ecosystems are far more complex than direct acute toxicity alone. For example, photoisomerization of dieldrin leads to the formation of a more toxic compound (Robinson *et al.*, 1966; Rosen *et al.*, 1966; Rosen and Sutherland, 1967) and details of the acute toxicity of this photoisomerization product to several species have been published (Brown *et al.*, 1967a; Wiese *et al.*, 1973).

Predictive toxicity tests for pesticides in relation to domesticated animals are generally less difficult than for wild animals as the actual target species can generally be used as the test model. For example, the use of ectoparasiticides can be tested on relatively small numbers of the host

33

34

species of interest without the necessity to use either valuable pedigree animals or large numbers of animals (Khan and Haufe, 1972; Ivey et al., 1972; Khan, 1973; Machin et al., 1974).

The use of laboratory animals to assess toxicity to man is common practice (Barnes, 1953; Frazer and Sharratt, 1969; Weil, 1972a and 1972b; Dixon, 1976; Krasovskij, 1976). Such extrapolation of data requires extreme caution and this has been expressed in a picturesque way by Schneiderman et al. (1975): 'When we extrapolate moderate or high dose animal toxicity to presumed effects in man, we must do it like the animal trainer entering the lion's cage—very cautiously.'

A clear demonstration of the difficulties of extrapolation of toxicity data from one species to another is found in published studies on fenclozic acid, an experimental anti-inflammatory drug (Alcock, 1971). No adverse effects were elicited by the compound in mouse (neo-natal and adult); rat (neo-natal and adult); dog; Rhesus monkey; Patas monkey; rabbit; guinea-pig; ferret; cat; pig; cattle; horse, but fenclozic acid caused acute cholestatic jaundice in man. Fenclozic acid is not a pesticide but it is included here because it is such a superb example of the outcome of acute exposure in man differing from that in a wide range of animal species.

Although pesticides are sometimes administered to humans for investigative purposes the legal and moral issues are somewhat different from those experienced when testing new medicinal products.[a] Acute toxicity tests carried out in man are generally at doses that are low when compared with the lethal doses predicted from animal experiments. The design of acute toxicity tests utilizing humans is generally based on the assessment of measurable changes in the blood chemistry, changes in other measurable physiological variables and the assay of the toxicant and its metabolites in the blood, other tissues and excreta (Wills et al., 1968; Nosal and Hladka, 1968; Rider et al., 1969). With pesticides useful human data on acute toxicology have often been obtained by the study of adventitiously exposed subjects (Jager, 1970; Jager et al., 1970; Radomski et al., 1971; Davies and Edmundson, 1972; Copplestone et al., 1976).

AVAILABILITY OF TEST SPECIES

The sub-kingdom of vertebrate animals is numerically very large and may be divided into distinct categories each containing many species (Table 3.1). Only a few of these species could be described as being at risk from the acute toxic properties of pesticides. However, there are indirect adverse effects attributable to pesticides upsetting the ecosystem and hence producing apparent acute effects on animals. For example, fish may be killed by oxygen depletion in the water because herbicides have been used

[a]See for example 'Experiments and Research with Humans: Values in Conflict'. Academy Forum, 3rd in series, National Academy of Sciences, Washington D.C., 1975.

Table 3.1 Approximate distribution of
the vertebrate animals (Rothschild, 1961)

Category	No. of different species (approximate)
Fish	23 000
Amphibians	2 000
Reptiles	8 500
Mammals	4 500
All vertebrates	43 000

for aquatic weed control although the herbicides used may not be very directly toxic to the fish (Newbold, 1975; Hurlbert, 1975).

For obvious practical reasons only a small number of the total animal species are available for test purposes (Schroeder, 1967), some of which are discussed below. Clearly not every species that has been used is discussed (Caldwell *et al.*, 1978) and it would not be helpful to create a long list of the rarer examples.

Mammals

Because of their size, breeding performance, ease of husbandry, and convenient life-span, some of the various rodent species have been developed into the most commonly used laboratory animals. Two rodent species are most often used for the study of acute toxicity, the laboratory rat (*Rattus norvegicus*) and the laboratory mouse (*Mus musculus*); it is doubtful whether any pesticide has been developed without its acute toxicity being assessed in one or both of these species. However, there are interesting perversities associated with the use of these two species. It might be assumed that these rodents would be ideal for studying the acute toxicities of rodenticides but the laboratory rat (*Rattus norvegicus*) responds very differently, in a quantitative sense, from the wild brown rat (*Rattus rattus*) to anticoagulant rodenticides (U.K. Ministry of Agriculture, Fisheries and Food, Pest Infestation Control Laboratory Technical Circular No. 26) but the acute toxicity of these anticoagulants is similar for man and for the brown rat (U.K. Ministry of Agriculture, Fisheries and Food, Pest Control Laboratory Technical Circular No. 29). Thus *Rattus norvegicus* is a poor model for predicting the rodenticidal properties of anticoagulants and also for predicting their acute toxicity to man. Roszkowski (1965), investigating the selective rodenticide norbormide determined the acute toxicity values for a wide range of species and found that rodents other than members of the family *Rattus* were resistant to intoxication as were non-rodents, in fact the cotton rat (*Sigmodon hispidus*) which, at least superficially, closely resembles the *Rattus norvegicus* was resistant to norbormide intoxication.

Norbormide

The laboratory mouse (*Mus musculus*) is commonly used for acute toxicity testing because of its convenient small size and ease of breeding and husbandry. There is a tendency for the mouse to be less susceptible to acute intoxication than the laboratory rat (*Rattus norvegicus*) but this is not invariably the case.

There are numerous other rodent species that are amenable to use for acute toxicity testing because they can be maintained easily in laboratories but various shortcomings may be found for each one. The Mongolian gerbil (*Meriones unguiculatus*) has a water metabolism that is adapted to desert life, hence its urine is highly concentrated and this may make the excretion of toxicants or metabolites unusual in relation to many other mammals (Rich, 1968) and it has been shown to be highly resistant to the lethal effects of irradiation (Chang *et al.*, 1964) and this may indicate some physiological peculiarity. Mertens *et al.* (1974 and 1975) have used the Mongolian gerbil for behavioural studies with the animals under the influence of pesticides. Steen *et al.* (1976) found that the acute toxicity of the organophosphate mevinphos to the Mongolian gerbil exhibited a sex difference that was the opposite of that found with rats exposed to the same compound (i.e. female rats are more susceptible to mevinphos intoxication than are male rats whereas the reverse is the case for the Mongolian gerbil).

The Syrian hamster (*Mesocricetus auratus*), the Chinese hamster (*Cricetulus griseus*) and the European hamster (*Cricetus cricetus*) have all been used in toxicity studies; however, the European hamster is uncommon as a laboratory animal (Farnsworth, 1977; Silverman and Chavannes, 1977) and the Chinese hamster is more often used for cytogenetic investigations than for acute toxicity testing. Since the Chinese hamster is a small rodent, about the same size as the laboratory mouse when fully grown, the species could be considered as a useful rodent for acute toxicity studies but it has a reputation for being difficult to breed (Hubble and Taylor, 1976). The Syrian hamster possesses a two-chambered stomach (Magalhaes, 1968) but generally responds to toxicants in a manner similar to the laboratory rat (*Rattus norvegicus*). The Syrian hamster has been shown to be much more sensitive to intoxication by both penicillin and strychnine than other rodents investigated (Wills, 1968), but it is a far less sensitive species than the mouse to intoxication by DDT (Agthe *et al.*, 1970; Truhaut *et al.*, 1974). This difference in sensitivity to DDT has been shown by Gingell and Wallcare (1974) to be due to significant differences in the concentration of toxicant in the brain (i.e. following identical exposures, the concentration of DDT in the brain of the mouse was twice as great as that in the brain of the Syrian hamster) and these investigators concluded that differences in the permeability of the respective blood–brain barriers might be the explanation. Truhaut *et al.* (1974) have shown that the Syrian hamster is generally much less sensitive to acute intoxication by the chlorinated hydrocarbon insecticides than are either rats or mice (Table 3.2).

The collard lemming (*Dicrostonyx stevensonii*, Nelson) has been used for some biomedical research (Dietrich, 1975). This species has not yet been exploited for toxicological studies but its very high basal metabolic rate is likely to make it of interest for some specialist studies.

Absence of a centrally motivated vomit reflex is characteristic of many rodents (Borison and Wang, 1953) and this has the advantage in experimental toxicology that once a toxicant has been instilled into the stomach the rodent cannot expel it. The guinea-pig (*Cavia porcellus*) is a rodent that can effectively regurgitate stomach contents and the species also differs from other commonly used rodents, but is similar to the rabbit, in being a caecal herbivore.

Closely related to the rodents are the lagomorphs. The rabbit (*Oryctolagus cuniculus*) is a member of that class and commonly used in predictive acute toxicity tests. In particular the rabbit is used in the

Table 3.2 The acute oral toxicities of some organochlorine pesticides to mice, rats, and Syrian hamsters. All pesticides administered as solutions in olive oil with a standard dosage of 2 ml/100 g bodyweight (Data from Truhaut *et al.*, 1974)

	LD_{50} mg/kg		
	Mouse (CF No. 1 strain) 30–35 g	Rat (Wistar Afhan strain) 250–285 g	Syrian hamster (strain not stated) 80–110 g
DDT (tech)	200 ± 16	215 ± 13	>10 000
pp′DDT	110 ± 13	120 ± 12	>5 000
DDD	3 500 ± 243	3 750 ± 280	>5 000
Chlordane	390 ± 35	350 ± 22	1 720 ± 135
Heptachlor	70 ± 7	105 ± 12	100 ± 11
Dieldrin	40 ± 3	45 ± 3	330 ± 45
Aldrin	45 ± 3	37.5 ± 5	320 ± 30
Lindane	90 ± 8	100 ± 9	360 ± 45
Endosulphan	85 ± 5	64 ± 4	118 ± 16

assessment of percutaneous toxicity (Draize, 1959; Draize *et al.*, 1944; Shah and Guthrie, 1977) although the rationale for this choice of test species is weak (Brown V. K. H., 1965 and 1966). The rabbit is not generally considered to be a good model for predicting the acute toxicity of products to other species by the oral route as it is a caecal herbivore (Hörnicke, 1977) and it has been demonstrated that fasting so prolongs gastric emptying that absorption from the gastro-intestinal tract is severely affected; however, Maeda *et al.* (1977) have developed a technique for using the rabbit for pharmacokinetic studies on gastro-intestinal absorption and this model has been demonstrated in their experiments as correlating well with bioavailability measurements in humans.

A commonly used non-rodent and non-lagomorph species for the laboratory assessment of the acute toxicity of pesticides is the dog (*Canis familiaris*). Unlike the rodents, dogs possess a highly developed vomit reflex and frequently are able to void all or part of any toxicant introduced into the alimentary tract before absorption can be completed. Generally the dog is not exceptional in its response to acute intoxication by pesticides, but Hutson and Hathway (1967) found the dog to be remarkably insensitive to intoxication by the organophosphorus insecticide chlorfenvinphos.

Although the ferret (*Mustela putorius furo*) has long attracted attention as a laboratory species (Pyle, 1940), this carnivore has not achieved any significant status in acute toxicity testing.

Because the pig (*Sus scrofa*) has some physiological resemblance to man (Jolly, 1970), it might have been a useful species for acute toxicity studies designed to predict hazard to man. The pig has been used for a wide variety of medical research (Bustad and Burns, 1966) but the size of the species does not make for ease of handling in acute toxicity studies. The miniature pig has proved popular as a substitute for the conventional pig in some research (Bustad and Burns, 1966) but the term miniature is relative and it is still too large for other than occasional special acute toxicity investigations. As a model for skin penetration studies, particularly *in vitro* investigations, the pig has created interest (Tregear, 1964; McCreesh, 1965) but the limitations of the species for this purpose are discussed in Chapter 5.

The domestic cat (*Felis catus*) is generally used only for acute toxicity studies on pesticides that are intended for use in feline veterinary medicine or for the investigation of neuropathies associated with organomercurial intoxication (Grant, 1971) or with organophosphorus compounds (Aldridge *et al.*, 1969).

Matsushima and Abe (1974) suggested that primates should be usable for toxicity studies with pesticides because of their similarity to man. Following paraquat intoxication similar interstitial fibroses are formed in the lungs of monkeys and man (Murray and Gibson, 1972 and 1974; Witschi and Kacew, 1974) but monkeys are generally insensitive to fluoroacetate intoxication when compared to man (Peters, 1963; Hashimoto et al., 1968). Wester and Maibach (1975) have investigated percutaneous absorption using the skin of rhesus monkey in vivo and this is discussed in Chapter 5.

Wild mammals are sometimes used for specialized studies. These may be free-ranging feral animals as in the studies on the increased toxicity of dieldrin following exposure to sunlight on the grass of South Africa, in which Wiese et al. (1973) investigated toxicity to the antelopes. (Note: The use of dieldrin on pastures is not a recommended procedure.) Alternatively, the wild animals may be held captive, as for example in the studies of Blackmore (1963) with foxes exposed to dieldrin.

Domesticated and other economic animals are vulnerable to the effects of pesticides. These animals may be deliberately exposed to anthelmintics and ectoparasiticides or adventitiously exposed to other pesticides (Radeleff and Bushland, 1953; Radeleff, 1970; Clarke and Clarke, 1975; Buck, 1975; Johnson et al., 1975). Mostly predictive acute toxicity tests can be carried out with the target species thus avoiding the need for extrapolation of data from one species to another. For example, Mia et al. (1973) were able to study the toxicity of organophosphates to goats and assess their safety for use in farms in areas of the world in which the goat is an important economic animal and similarly Palmer and Schlinke (1973) investigated the toxicity of an organophosphorus defoliant to cattle and sheep. There is little or no merit in using economic animals for the prediction of toxicity to man.

An indication of the distribution of mammals used for acute toxicity testing with pesticides can be obtained by analysis of information contained in the World Health Organization review of carbamates and organophosphorus insecticides used in agriculture and public health (Vettorazzi and Miles-Vettorazzi, 1975). Details of 28 compounds are included in the review of published information and Table 3.3 indicates the

Table 3.3 The species used for a number of acute toxicity tests. (Data from Vettorazzi and Miles-Vettorazzi, 1975)

Species	No. of tests	No. of compounds
Cat	12	9
Cattle	6	6
Dog	23	19
Guinea-pig	39	28
Mouse	88	38
Rabbit	34	23
Rat	203	38
Other species	6	6

species used for acute toxicity tests, the number of tests reported, and the number of compounds associated with each species.

There can be little doubt that a similar pattern of species used would be found for other classes of pesticides.

The differences in sensitivity of different species of mammals to intoxication can be critical to hazard assessment. In some instances the investigation of biochemical mechanisms can give valuable leads in the interpretation of effects. In a definitive study involving the hepatic tissues from nine mammalian species, Whitehouse and Ecobichon (1975) investigated parathion desulphuration and arylesterase catalysed hydrolysis of paraoxon; taking into account the most sensitive sex for each species they found species differences in sensitivity as in Table 3.4.

These differences in sensitivity may, in part at least, account for some of the species differences recorded for the acute toxicity of parathion. Investigating another organophosphorus insecticide, chlorfenvinphos, Hutson and Hathway (1967) were able to account for the very large species differences in sensitivity to acute intoxication, in combined absorption–metabolism rate, and in the relative sensitivities of the brain cholinesterases of the two species to inhibition by the compound.

An analysis of data on the relative sensitivity of man and other mammals to acute intoxication by 260 chemicals has been published by Krasovskij (1975). Because of lack of clarity in the review, it must be assumed that the reviewer included variables of intoxication other than death. Krasovskij concluded that man was more sensitive than the other species tested in a large number of cases and for many chemicals as many as 11 other species were investigated. By selecting the rat as test animal and designating the acute toxicity in that species arbitrarily as one, sensitivity ratios for man were as shown in Table 3.5.

Table 3.4 Ranking of parathion desulphuration and paraoxon hydrolysis for hepatic tissue from different species. (Data from Whitehouse and Ecobichon, 1975)

Parathion desulphuration	Paraoxon hydrolysis
Most activity	
Syrian hamster	Mouse
Guinea-pig	Cattle
Mouse	Rat
Rat	Guinea-pig
Rabbit	Rabbit
Cattle	Syrian hamster
Dog	Cay
Pig	Dog
Cat	Pig
Least activity	

Table 3.5   Ratios of the sensitivities of man and rat to acute intoxication
by different classes of compounds. (Data from Krasovskij, 1975)

Chemical class	Number of compounds	Sensitivity ratio (man : rat when rat = 1)
Inorganic compounds	40	4.2 ± 0.66
Organophosphorus compounds	16	1.9 ± 0.46
Organochlorine compounds	20	1.8 ± 0.30
'Drugs'	62	10.5 ± 5.80

However, there were enormous differences within the responses to the different chemical classes (e.g. within the organophosphorus group a factor of nearly 50 could be applied).

Further, Krasovskij (1975) reviewed the sensitivity of different species to compounds and in this series it was found that the most sensitive species were:

Mouse	38 cases
Rabbit	28 cases
Dog	44 cases

These were in a total of 154 cases and the number of species investigated ranged from 3 to 6. In several instances there was more than one species at the most sensitive end of the scale. An important conclusion from this review by Krasovskij.is that primates are virtually indistinguishable from other laboratory animals in their sensitivity to acute intoxication by chemicals.

Birds

Many species of birds are vulnerable to intoxication by pesticides and generally this is undesirable. However, there are some species of birds that may be considered as pests and their susceptibility to the avicidal properties of chemicals may be considered an advantage.

Predictive acute toxicity tests are often carried out in the laboratory using captive birds and valuable information can be obtained from such studies, provided that possible differences between the responses in feral and the non-feral birds are taken into consideration (Brown V. K. H., 1974).

Many different avian species have been used in predictive acute toxicity testing (McFarland and Lacey, 1968; Tucker and Haegele, 1971; Schafer, 1972; Schafer and Cunningham, 1972; Schafer et al., 1973). Species differences in sensitivity to intoxication can be large. For example, the avicide, 3-chloro-p-toluidine is highly toxic to some birds and of a low order of toxicity to others and Felsenstein et al. (1974) demonstrated that in the more susceptible species of birds the mode of action is principally nephrotoxicity.

In another detailed study several pesticides were examined for their effects on six avian species. The investigators, Tucker and Haegele (1971), concluded that the extrapolation of data from one bird species to another was unrewarding. A review of the metabolism of chemicals by birds has been published by Pan and Fouts (1978).

Because of relative insensitivity to intoxication by many chemicals the domestic fowl (*Gallus domesticus*) is not generally regarded as a satisfactory laboratory species for predictive tests, although it has many advantages in terms of availability and ease of husbandry. For example, the veterinary anthelmintic haloxon has been shown to have an oral LD_{50} value of 50 mg/kg in geese but in domestic fowl the comparable figure is greater than 5 000 mg/kg (Lee and Pickering, 1967). The other avian species quite often used in laboratory investigations are the Japanese quail (*Corturnix corturnix japonica*) and the common pigeon (*Columba livia*). The Japanese quail has been recommended as the bird of choice for acute toxicity studies in the U.K. Pesticide Safety Precautions Scheme. Bunyan *et al.* (1971) reported that pigeons were significantly more susceptible to intoxication by chlorfenvinphos than were pheasants or Japanese quail. These investigators attributed this observation to the differential inhibition of the brain isoesterases in pigeons not observed in the other two species.

Something of the limitation on species extrapolation among birds can be seen with the available data on carbophenothion which caused a massive kill of Greylag geese in Scotland when applied as a seed-dressing (Jennings *et al.*, 1975); the acute oral toxicity values for carbophenothion in birds are shown in Table 3.6.

Birds cannot generally be used as an indicator of acute toxic hazard for mammals. An important exception is the use of some bird species to investigate the neuropathies associated with acute exposure to certain classes of compounds. The adult domestic fowl (*Gallus domesticus*) is an excellent indicator of the type of delayed neurotoxicity associated with acute exposure to some organophosphates (Aldridge *et al.*, 1969; Albert and Stearns, 1974), whereas many mammals are resistant to this effect

Table 3.6 The acute oral toxicity of carbophenothion to some bird species.

Species	LD_{50} value (mg/kg)	Source
Starlings	5.6	Schafer, 1972
Redwings	7.5	Schafer, 1972
Pigeons	34.8 (31.1–38.9)	Jennings *et al.*, 1975
Japanese quail	56.8 (50.8–63.6)	Jennings *et al.*, 1975
Canada geese	29 to 35	Jennings *et al.*, 1975
Mallards	121 (95.9–152)	Tucker and Crabtree, 1970
Domestic fowl	316	Jennings *et al.*, 1975

(Majno and Karnovsky, 1961). The Pekin duck (*Anas platorhynchos*, var.) has been used to study the aetiology of the spongy degeneration of the white matter caused by some toxicants (Carlton and Kreutzberg, 1966; Carlton, 1967). Revzin (1976a) has used pigeons to investigate the effect of cholinesterase inhibitors on memory and concentration.

Fish

Fish may be exposed to pesticides because of the deliberate addition of pesticides to the water (e.g. herbicides for aquatic weed control, insecticides for malaria eradication, molluscicides for bilharzia controls, etc.) or because of adventitious contamination (e.g. insecticide spray drift, washing out of contaminated containers and equipment, emptying of cattle and sheep dip baths, etc.). On occasions pesticides may even be used deliberately because of their piscicidal properties such as the use of rotenone to kill edible fish in some parts of the world.

The piscicidal properties of pesticides can be examined in the laboratory (Mawdesley-Thomas *et al.*, 1974). Most of these studies are made with fresh-water species (Cope, 1961, 1964, and 1965; Hughes and Davis, 1963; Alabaster, 1969a and 1969b; Muirhead-Thomson, 1971; Reiff, 1974), less often with estuarine fish (Butler, 1965) and even less frequently with sea fish (Holden, 1973; Baba *et al.*, 1976). This pattern of priorities for investigations follows the overall likelihood of exposure occurring (Mawdesley-Thomas, 1971; Bathe *et al.*, 1974).

Ideally fish toxicity tests are carried out under natural conditions but most predictive acute toxicity tests have to be carried out in aquariums. Essentially predictive toxicity tests with fish may take one of three forms:

(i) Static method

These are simple tests and are generally inaccurate. Water containing appropriate concentrations of the pesticide is placed in aquariums together with the test fish. Signs of toxication and mortality are recorded for a period of time. The test method takes no account of diminution in concentration of pesticide with time (i.e. due to uptake by fish, adsorption on to vessel surface, breakdown and other losses) nor to the accumulation of excretion products, possibly including toxic metabolites, from the fish.

(ii) Semi-dynamic method

This method is slightly advantageous over method (i) in that at regular intervals a portion of the water is removed from the aquariums and is replaced by an equal volume of water containing the required concentration of toxicants. This method is favoured by the United Kingdom Pesticide Safety Precaution Scheme and may easily be automated (Alabaster, 1969a and 1969b).

(iii) Dynamic method.

This is the most useful test method but one that is difficult to carry out and uses a relatively large amount of pesticide when compared with methods (i) and (ii). The test fish are kept in aquariums with the water containing the pesticide flowing in from a source and constantly being removed by means of an overflow, thus the concentration of toxicant is kept approximately constant throughout the exposure period and all excretion and breakdown products are removed.

For all three test methods it is desirable to monitor the concentrations of toxicant throughout the exposure period.

None of the three test methods takes into account the indirect toxicity of pesticides to fish that may be brought about by such mechanism as deoxygenation due to the destruction of aquatic flora or the upset of the food balance by the killing of the micro-fauna.

Since the water represents to fish an atmosphere that may be compared, in some ways, with the air surrounding the terrestial vertebrates, it might be possible to apply Haber's rule (see Chapter 5) that the effect of the multiple of time of exposure and concentration is constant. As with inhalation exposure in terrestrial vertebrates this is only approximately correct and data handled in this way must be considered with caution.

In the design and performance of predictive tests for the acute toxicity of pesticides to fish it is essential to take into account the absolute size of the fish, the relationship between the size of the fish and the volume of the water, and the temperature of the water in the aquariums in relation to the species of fish used. Generally the volume of water containing toxicant must be very large in relation to the volume of fish used.

As with mammals and birds, there can be enormous species differences in susceptibility of fish to intoxication (Gibson, 1977). Fish of different ages may respond differently to the same toxicant and in order to assess the hazard to the new-born it must be recalled that some fish lay eggs and others are viviparous.

There is no single correlation between toxicity to fish and toxicity to mammals (Bathe *et al.*, 1976) although it is sometimes possible to make predictions based on known metabolic patterns. For example, Benke *et al.*

Table 3.7 The relative acute toxicities of two pesticides to a fish species and to a mammalian species. (Data from Benke *et al.*, 1974.)

Toxicant	LD_{50} (mg/kg)	
	Sunfish	Mouse
Methylparathion	>2 500	11.0 ± 0.8
Parathion	110 ± 67	13.5 ± 1.3

(1974) demonstrated that parathion and methylparathion have similar LD_{50} values in mice but that in the sunfish (*Lepomis gibbosus*) the acute toxicity values are quite different (Table 3.7); the investigators explained this phenomenon as being due to slower death in the fish which favours GSH-dependent and also hydrolytic-dependent degradation of methylparathion.

Reptiles

Apart from efforts to conserve the ecological balance, reptiles are not generally considered worthy of much concern. Largely because of pesticide use-patterns reptiles are not generally very vulnerable to intoxication and for this reason rarely feature in programmes of predictive acute toxicity testing.

Amphibians

Amphibians are obviously vulnerable to pesticide intoxication in water or on land (Edery and Schatzberg-Porath, 1960). The general principles of exposure in the aquatic environment are similar to those for fish although it must not be assumed that fish and amphibia will respond in the same way to a toxicant for their physiology is very different. On land amphibians are frequently to be found in the more shaded and often damp regions and they may be affected by pesticides used to treat the area (Kaplan and Overpeck, 1964).

Frogs and toads at all stages of development are amenable to use for predictive tests in the laboratory (Cooke, 1972; Nishiuchi and Yoshida, 1974).

STATUS OF THE TEST ANIMAL

It is a truism that the major purpose of most acute toxicity testing is to predict hazard. The response of any animal, including man, to a toxicant is associated with the biological physical status of the target animal. Therefore to compensate for the biological and physical variants when making the predictions, acute toxicity tests are generally orientated to population risks rather than to individual responses (Waud, 1972) for individuals do not necessarily behave in mathematically predictable terms.

Each individual in any biological group differs in some way from all other members of the group even though the differences may be very small in some cases. For predictive toxicity testing the trend is to utilize homogeneous animal populations and then to maintain them under near ideal conditions before and during the exposure to the toxicant.

Physiological bias can easily be introduced into the animal population by methods of husbandry and this in turn may introduce changes in sensitivity to the affects of toxicants (Brown, A. M., 1961, 1964, and 1965; Guthrie *et al.*, 1971; National Academy of Sciences, 1971). Conversely, as a species man is extremely heterogeneous and as a target for toxic reaction is affected by ethnic differences, disease status, social conditions, etc. Pharmacogenetic variability is commonplace in man and in many other species (Kalow, 1962 and 1965; Meier, 1963).

The presence or absence of even qualitative differences in enzyme systems may account for variation in the responses observed with the same toxicant in different apparently closely related species. This has been demonstrated for the influence of cytochrome P-450 on several substrates in various animal species by Flynn *et al.* (1972). Litterst *et al.* (1975) investigated microsomal and soluble-fraction enzymes from the lungs, liver, and kidneys of rat, mouse, rabbit, Syrian hamster, and guinea pig and found that no species demonstrated total superiority in drug-metabolizing activity; in many estimations the Syrian hamster was shown to be best and the rat was surprisingly poor. The same investigators (Litterst *et al.*, 1975) found that the mouse exhibited glutathione-*S*-aryltransferase activity in the lungs and kidneys that was up to ten times greater than that in any other species in their investigation and that this level of activity was comparable with the activities in the livers of rabbit and guinea-pig. Other physiological differences such as the acid content of the stomachs of different species can change the bioavailability of some toxicants (Smyth, 1964) and the flora of the intestinal tract can cause differences in response in different species and even between individuals within a species (Scheline, 1968; Smith, 1971).

Many other factors may seriously affect the status of the test animal and some of these are discussed below:

Size

The results of acute toxicity tests are generally expressed in terms of either bodyweight or body surface-area and, of these two, bodyweight is the more commonly used. Hart (1967) stated that the most common dose to bodyweight relationship is a direct linear function characterized by a slope of unity when plotted as a graph. However, Hart (1967) and Lamanna and Hart (1968) went on to demonstrate that in a significant number of examples the character of the response may vary with the toxicant, with its route of administration, and also with the sex of the exposed animal. In addition, other factors such as the strain of test animal are known to alter the responses observed in mice, rats, Syrian hamsters, dogs, and monkeys, species, Hart (1967) and Lamanna and Hart (1968) included only two pesticides, sodium fluoroacetate and alphanaphthylthiourea and of these two the intraperitoneal toxicity of sodium fluoroacetate deviated from linearity when administered to female mice.

In a published review Paget and Barnes (1964) indicated that the extrapolation of acute toxicity data from small animals to man on the basis of relative bodyweights could give rise to ratios that are as much as ten times greater than if the same extrapolations are based on body surface-area ratios.

Utilizing information about anti-cancer drugs from which it is possible to make accurate comparisons between the responses observed in man and the responses observed in mice, rats, Syrian hamsters, dogs, and monkeys, the research and clinical investigators Freireich *et al.* (1966) found a better correlation between the response and the body surface-area rather than that between the response and the bodyweight. These investigators emphasized that there are intrinsic dangers in extrapolating results directly from animals to man and that calculations of dosage based on body surface-area do not have automatic merit.

Angelakos (1960) found that there are toxicants that in some species generate data that defy relationship between either bodyweight or body surface-area and dose. Rall and North (1953) investigated the acute toxicity of the rodenticide alphanaphthylthiourea in wild Norway rats and found that a log-log plot of the LD_{50} values against the bodyweights of the animals gave rise to a linear dose–response line, but if these data are compared with the data obtained for the same compound in mice (Lamanna and Hart, 1968), slopes of the graphs are found to be inverted; Rall and North (1953) suggested that the actual relationship could best be expressed in terms of dose per animal.

Within reasonable limits body surface-area may be considered to be a function of bodyweight and this function is expressed by the equation: when

$$A = k \cdot W^x$$

A = body surface-area (cm^2)

W = bodyweight (g)

k and x = variables for different species

Values for k and x have been published for many species (Spector, 1956; Holliday *et al.*, 1967). However, there are many other physiological functions (F) that might be related to bodyweight by the general formula: when

$$F = k_s \cdot W^y$$

F = specified function

k_s = constant for specified function

y = constant for specified function

W = bodyweight (g)

Derome (1977) has provided a rigorous mathematical analysis of these allometric equations using group and similarity theory. In an earlier detailed analysis of the subject, Zeuthen (1953) showed that this formula can be applied logically to the relationship between oxygen uptake and body size in all organisms, thus it is possible to define the function (F) as the 'metabolic bodyweight'. Thonney *et al*. (1974) found that there are highly significant differences between the sexes for the 'metabolic bodyweights' in a number of animal species.

Although some acute toxicity data may be capable of relation to bodyweight by the use of this equation, the inherent danger of false correlation has been documented (Adolph, 1949; Tanner, 1949; Brody, 1964).

The relationship for the values of the slopes of oxygen uptake plotted against body size has been shown to be simple and consistent for all animals from the unicellular to higher advanced multicellular (Zeuthen, 1953). Furthermore, if plots are made during the development of the multicellular animal, that is as size increases from egg to adult, the same family of curves is obtained and this is called 'ontogenetic recapitulation'. This relationship does not apply to acute toxicity data.

Krebs (1950) demonstrated that the characteristic differences in the basal rate of heat production in animals of differing sizes are attributable to the oxygen quotient of the musculature. The oxygen quotients of tissues other than muscle are governed by the specific heat requirements of the tissues and not by the heat requirement of the whole body. On the basis that metabolic rate is not directly proportional to bodyweight, Kleiber (1975) has been critical of the term 'metabolic bodyweight'. The basis for Kleiber's criticism lies in the fact that heat flow per unit of bodyweight has no proper physical or physiological meaning. Earlier, von Bertalanffy (1951) distinguished between metabolic types in respect of the metabolic rate and the body size and he put both fish and mammals into one group with the general group title 'respiration surface proportional', because either they exhibited a linear growth curve without inflexion or else they exhibited a sigmoid weight–growth curve.

Table 3.8 is a reproduction of a table published by Lehman (1959) concerning the relationship of drug toxicity in experimental animals compared to man. No correlation can be attributed to dose and bodyweight nor to dose and body surface-area with these data.

Krasovskij (1975) found a linear relationship between many physiological functions and bodyweight in a wide range of mammalian species. His range of correlations included such diverse functions as longevity, microsomal enzyme activities, relative organ weights, pulse, and respiration rates; the only serious exception to this finding was the differential leucocyte counts which did not correlate with bodyweight. Krasovskij compared the logarithms of the lethal doses of 278 substances (N.B. stated to belong to 7 different groups of chemical types—but the groups were not listed) against the logarithms of the bodyweights of between 6 and 10 different animal species (N.B. again no list). Further

Table 3.8 Some relations of drug toxicity in experimental animals compared to man*. (Data from Lehman, 1959.)

Animal	Weight (kg)	Weight ratio animal/man	Drug dose ratio animal/man	Sensitivity Drug dose ratio/weight ratio
Man	60	1	1	1
Cow	500	8	24	Man is 3 times as sensitive
Horse	500	8	16	Man is 2 times as sensitive
Sheep	60	1	3	Man is 3 times as sensitive
Goat	60	1	3	Man is 3 times as sensitive
Swine	60	1	2	Man is 2 times as sensitive
Dog	10	1/6	1	Man is 6 times as sensitive
Cat	3	1/20	1/2	Man is 10 times as sensitive
Rat	0.4	1/150	1/15	Man is 10 times as sensitive

*The values in this table are averages and their origins cannot be checked as Lehman (1959) only recorded them as being from numerous sources.

correlations were made for the pharmacological action of 238 drugs, from 6 unspecified groups, using 7 to 10 mammalian species; both sets of data showed very good correlation. The coefficient of correlation for the former was 0.60–0.92 (slope β = 0.62–0.81) and the coefficient of correlation for the latter was 0.81–0.94 (slope β = 0.52–0.69).

Krasovskij (1975) suggested a general rule called the 'determining principle of bodyweight'. This rule may be expressed as: The logarithms of the biological parameters of mammals are linear functions of the logarithms of bodyweight. He carried out regression analysis on the acute toxicity data for over 400 chemicals and on pharmacological response to about 250 compounds and found that the 'determining principle of bodyweight' was applicable to between 80 and 85% of his examples. For the remaining 15 to 20% it was necessary to consider allometric relationships (i.e. disproportionate relationships between biological parameter and bodyweight), however, unfortunately Krasovskij has not revealed detailed findings with these data.

For toxicants that are dependent on altering the susceptibility of the intoxicated animal to its environment (e.g. changes in sensitivity to the ambient temperature), it is more probable that the body surface-area will be critical rather than the bodyweight within the species. Cornwell and Bull (1967) demonstrated that this was the case for the rodenticide alphachloralose.

Funaki (1974), working with mice, rats, rabbits, dogs, and humans, measured body surface-areas (S) cm², body length (H) cm, bodyweights (W) g and found that the logarithm of the bodyweight was linearly related to the logarithm of the body length:

$$H = 3.31\ W^{0.335}$$

and body length was linearly related to the logarithm of the body surface-area:

$$S = 1.39 \, H^{1.83}$$

These two equations may be transformed to:

$$S = 10.4 \, W^{0.667}$$

which agrees with the generally accepted form:

$$S = k \, W^{2/3}$$

Studying the toxicity of several compounds and expressing the findings as LD_{50} values in mg/kg or mg/cm^2 or mol/cm^2, Funaki found no linear relation between the LD_{50} values in mg/kg and the values of W or log W, but there was a positive linear relationship between log LD_{50} in mg/cm^2 and S; also there was a negative linear relationship between log LD_{50} in mg/s and s, when

$$s = \frac{S}{W}$$

With a limited number of toxicants, Funaki (1974) went on to show that:

$$\text{bodyweight (kg)} \times LD_{50} \text{ (mg/kg)} = 0.001 \, 23 \, b \, W^{0.953} \qquad \text{(i)}$$

$$\text{bodyweight (kg)} \times LD_{50} \text{ (mg/kg)} = 0.002 \, 75 \, b \, W^{0.836} \qquad \text{(ii)}$$

when (i) is intravenous route, (ii) is oral route, and b is a constant and further,

$$\log [\text{bodyweight (kg)} \times LD_{50} \text{ (mg/kg)}] = k_1 \log S - k_2 \log W$$

when k_1 is the metabolic assimilation velocity constant
and k_2 is the metabolic dissimilation velocity constant

$$k_1 \, \Sigma(\log S)^2 - k_2 \, \Sigma \log S \cdot \log W =$$
$$\Sigma \log[\text{bodyweight (kg)} \times LD_{50} \text{ (mg/kg)}] \times \log S$$

$$k_1 \, \Sigma \log S \cdot \log W - k_2 \, \Sigma(\log W)^2 =$$
$$\Sigma \log[\text{bodyweight (kg)} \times LD_{50} \text{ (mg/kg)}] \times \log W$$

Dedrick (1974) has put the problem of scaling-up from one species to another into sharp perspective. He has pointed out that there are only five orders of magnitude separating the bodyweights of a mouse and an elephant whereas there are more than eight orders of magnitude separating the bodyweight of a typical mouse and that of a typical cell and also there are more than twelve orders of magnitude separating the weight of a typical cell and that of a typical protein molecule. Each of these parameters is involved in the pharmacokinetic extrapolation from one species to another. Many other variables also affect the toxicological response, for example overt changes in body composition such as changes in the fat distribution (Lesser *et al.*, 1973). Species variation in basal metabolic rate is well known and can influence the validity of any scaling-up; Dieterich (1975) found that the collared lemming (*Dicrostonyx stevensonii*, Nelson), although a rodent, has a basal metabolic rate at 25 to 30 °C that is about 40% greater than the expected value for other rodents of a similar size.

Predictably, in the total body exposure situation, such as the exposure of fish to toxicants in the water, the size of the exposed animals can affect uptake (Murphy, 1971). Because of the greater exposed area the larger animal may be differently at risk than smaller animals of the same species. Anderson and Weber (1975) investigated the influence of body size in relation to lethal concentrations of several toxicants to guppies (*Poecilia reticulata*) and concluded that relative measures of toxic potency at different animal sizes may be derived from the formula attributed to Bliss:

when

$$Y = a + b \log(M/W^h)$$

Y = per cent mortality expressed as Probit
M = mean toxicant concentration
W = weight of exposed animals
h = exponent of the function weight
a = intercept on the ordinate
b = slope of graph

or from the equation:

$$LD_{50} = \log a + b \log W$$

Anderson and Weber showed that the general formula:

$$LD_{50} = xW^h$$

can be applied when x is the abscissal value of log (M/W^h) corresponding to the 50% response level. The values of h obtained by Anderson and Weber (1975) varied greatly depending on the toxicant tested.

Age

Age variation may give rise to differences in susceptibility to acute intoxication by different toxicants and there is no simple rule for relating age to toxic response (Goldenthal, 1971; Hänninen, 1975).

Substantial differences in susceptibility to intoxication can sometimes be related to small age differences. With rats a few months' difference in age can profoundly affect the response to some chemicals that influence the central nervous system (Saunders *et al.*, 1974).

Biological ageing is both time- and species-dependent (Mann, Jr. 1965). For the purposes of toxicology and posology it is convenient to consider the biological ages as being neo-natal, infant, young adult, adult, and old, but there is no clear demarcation between these categories because development is a continuum. However, for some species, such as the rat, there is a linear relationship between the logarithm of the bodyweight and the reciprocal of the animal's age (Gray and Addis, 1948); this relationship may be expressed as:

$$Log_{10}(\text{bodyweight in grams}) = \frac{-k}{d} + log_{10}A$$

when,

k = slope of line

d = age in days

A = estimated asymptote or limit approached by the bodyweight.

Toxicological response to endogenous physiological chemicals (e.g. adrenalin, noradrenalin and acetylcholine) may vary with age. Brus and Herman (1971) demonstrated that new-born mice are significantly less sensitive to intoxication with adrenalin or noradrenalin than are adult mice but that the reverse holds good for acetylcholine. It has been suggested that this might reflect development of the cholinergic system in the species rather than metabolic differences. Studying developmental pharmacology in rats, Naik *et al.* (1970) found that brain acetylcholine concentration increased with bodyweight until maturity whereas the brain cholinesterase activity was variable at lower bodyweight and became more stable as weight and age increased. To obtain meaningful data on the influence of age on brain cholinesterase in man would be difficult, but Shanor *et al.* (1961) using a large population sample of young adults (age range 18–35 years) and older people (age range 70–80 years) found that the plasma cholinesterase activity was approximately 24% higher in the young males than in the old males; no plasma cholinesterase differences were found between young adult and old females and no differences were found between the age groups of either sex when erythrocyte cholinesterase was measured.

Freedman and Himwich (1948) studied the toxicity of the anticholinesterase agent di-isopropylfluorophosphate and demonstrated that neo-natal rats were more sensitive than rats aged a few days and that the sensitivity to intoxication diminished with further increase in age. A comparison of the acute toxicities of 16 anticholinesterase pesticides, 15 organophosphorus compounds, and 1 carbamate, to weanling and adult rats was made by Brodeur and DuBois (1963). When their data were translated into ratios of the mean LD_{50} values for weanling and for adult rats, of the 16 compounds only 4 were more toxic to weanlings than to adults and only with 1 compound did the reverse apply (Table 3.9). From the known metabolic pathways for these compounds (DuBois, 1971); Vandekar *et al.*, 1971; Dauterman, 1971) it is more probable that the

Table 3.9   Ratios of mean LD_{50} values for adult and weanling male rats. (Data from Brodeur and DuBois, 1963)

Compound	Ratio adult LD_{50}/weanling LD_{50}
Ethyl nitrophenyl-benzene thionophosphonate (EPN)	Greater than 3
Trithion	Greater than 3
Parathion	2–3
Malathion	2–3
Methylparathion	1–2
Systox	1–2
Di-syston	1–2
Ethion	1–2
Gluthion	1–2
Delnav	1–2
Phosdrin	1–2
Folex	1–2
Dipterex	1–2
Sevin	1–2
CO-RAL	1
Octamethyl pyrophosphoramide (OMPA)	Less than 1

differences can be attributed to the development of metabolizing enzymes as an age-dependent factor rather than to differential cholinesterase patterns. The fact that the one exception, octamethyl pyrophosphoramide, has been shown not to depress microsomal activity may be an important factor in the age-dependent sensitivity to the acute toxicities of the products (Stevens *et al.*, 1972).

During the study of age differences in the toxic response to parathion and methylparathion in rats, Benke and Murphy (1975) demonstrated that the age sensitivity differences were directly correlated with the metabolism of paraoxon and methylparaoxon rather than with cholinesterase inhibiting effects or other factors associated with the parent compounds. Harbison and Koshakji (1975) observed that the new-born rat was about five times more susceptible to intoxication by parathion than were the adult rats. However in their tests with rat liver microsomes the conversion from parathion into the oxygen analogue increased with increase in age and reached adult rates at about 30 days *post-partum*. These investigators concluded that the age-linked sensitivity could be attributed to a combination of depressed paraoxonase activity and a depressed cholinesterase activity in the new-born. These findings agree with the previous report of Brodeur and DuBois (1967) that the enzyme for the degradation of malathion (i.e. the enzyme responsible for the conversion of malathion into its oxygen analogue, malaoxon) is deficient in new-born and immature rats. More recently, Mendoza and Shields (1977) found that the LD_{50} values for malathion increased over the range of age from 209 mg/kg at 1 day to 1 806 mg/kg at 17 days; they observed excellent correlation

(correlation coefficient $= 0.099\ 65$) between the LD_{50} values for the age range and the I_{50} values for the brain cholinesterase in rats. Harbison (1975) confirmed the finding for parathion and its conversion to paraoxon and also demonstrated that adult male rats are more sensitive than new-born rats to DDT (approximately 10 times), chlordane (approximately 3 times), and heptachlor (approximately 7 times).

$$(MeO)_2 P.S.CH.\overset{\overset{\displaystyle O}{\|}}{C}OEt$$
$$\overset{\|}{S}\quad \overset{|}{C}H_2\underset{\underset{\displaystyle O}{\|}}{C}OEt$$

Malathion

$$(MeO)_2 P.S.CH.\overset{\overset{\displaystyle O}{\|}}{C}OEt$$
$$\overset{\|}{O}\quad \overset{|}{C}H_2\underset{\underset{\displaystyle O}{\|}}{C}OEt$$

Malaoxon

$$(EtO)_2 \overset{\overset{\displaystyle S}{\|}}{P}.O\!-\!\!\left\langle\!\!\bigcirc\!\!\right\rangle\!\!-NO_2$$

Parathion

$$(EtO)_2 \overset{\overset{\displaystyle O}{\|}}{P}.O\!-\!\!\left\langle\!\!\bigcirc\!\!\right\rangle\!\!-NO_2$$

Paraoxon

The metabolizing activity of the liver microsomal enzymes from rats varies from very little in the new-born to a maximum at 30 days, thereafter there is a decrease in the activity such that at 150 days it is only about half of that at 30 days (Kato et al., 1964) but, because of other susceptibility factors, the in vivo acute response may not exactly correlate for most compounds.

In a different study, but using rats, Lu et al. (1965) confirmed the finding of Brodeur and DuBois (1963) that malathion is significantly more toxic to young rats than to adult rats and they further demonstrated that neo-natal rats were even more sensitive that were weanlings. The same investigators also studied the acute toxicities of the chlorinated hydrocarbon pesticides DDT and dieldrin in the same age range rats, and concluded that the neo-natal rat is much less sensitive than either weanlings or adults to acute intoxication by these two compounds.

Interpretation of results in the neo-natal animal must not be confounded by information obtained from studies with animals exposed during the pre-natal period, since at this stage of development quantitative aspects of the metabolized enzyme systems may be severely altered (Khera and Clegg, 1969); indeed Jondorf et al. (1958) demonstrated that new-born mice and guinea-pigs lack enzymic mechanisms for metabolizing several compounds (e.g. monomethyl-4-aminoantipyrine, amidopyrine, phenacetin, hexobarbitone, etc.). Also these neo-natal animals are unable to form glucuronides as metabolites, but both of these metabolic mechanisms begin to appear in the first week of post-natal life and increase to a maximum at about eight weeks old.

Investigating the effects of drugs in new-born rats, Yeary et al. (1966)

and Yeary (1967) reported that the effects of maturation on acute toxicity was generally consistent within a pharmacological class of compounds but that there was no reason to suppose that new-born animals would be more sensitive than adults in all cases. The same conclusion was reached by Hudson *et al.* (1972) when they investigated the acute toxicities of 14 pesticides to mallard ducks at different ages.

Sodium fluoride, sometimes used for killing cockroaches and also as an anthelmintic for use in swine, has been shown by Mörnstad (1975) to be age-dependent in its acute toxicity to rats; this has been confirmed by De Lopez *et al.* (1976) and these latter investigators compared their findings on F^- content of the plasma with earlier data of Maynard (Table 3.10), and

Table 3.10(a) The acute intraperitoneal toxicity to rats of different ages exposed to sodium fluoride (Data from Mörnstad, 1975)

Age of animals (days)	LD_{50} values (mg/kg of F^-)	
	Male	Female
4	40 (34–48)	45 (39–52)
20	51 (47–55)	47 (39–57)
60	28 (17–42)	30 (21–43)
90	20 (17–24)	21 (17–26)

(b) The acute intraperitoneal toxicity to rats of different weights exposed to sodium fluoride (Data of Maynard quoted by De Lopez *et al.*, 1976)

Weight of animals (g)	LD_{50} values (mg/kg of F^-)
100–200	21
200–300	11

(c) The acute oral toxicity to rats of different weights exposed to sodium fluoride (Data from De Lopez *et al.*, 1976)

Weight of animals (g)	LD_{50} values (mg/kg of NaF) (95% confidence limits)
80	54 (49–54*)
150	52 (48–57)
250	31 (25–38)

*This figure appeared in the published paper but may have been a typographical error.

c

suggested that the age differences in susceptibility may be associated with uptake of F^- by bone. This age effect has also been demonstrated in relation to the susceptibility of carp to this compound (Neuhold and Sigler, 1960).

The pattern of distribution of toxicant in the body may vary with age. In particular the blood–brain barrier may not be functional in the neo-natal animal and the ability of some toxicants to accumulate in the brain may be correlated with the age-dependent development of the barrier (Kupferberg and Way, 1963). An indication that binding at sites may also be important has been provided by James and Kanungo (1976), these investigators also demonstrated that the acetylcholinesterase activity exhibited corresponding changes with age in rats.

An example of retrospective confirmation of a toxicological observation has been provided by Hanig et al. (1976). These investigators followed up the reports that a 1% preparation of lindane could be used safely for the treatment of scabies in adult humans but could cause convulsions and near fatality in children on a dose per bodyweight basis. Hanig et al. demonstrated that the toxic effects of the lindane formulation were minimal when applied to the skin of adult rabbits but that it caused convulsions and sometimes death in young (6 week old) rabbits, this being due to the relative rates of absorption and the age-linked differences in sensitivity to intoxication.

Ageing factors have been studied in depth in man and in other animals (Lasagna, 1956; Nyhan, 1961; Done, 1964; Stave, 1964; Litchfield, 1967; Hommes and Wilmink, 1968) and the conclusion remains that there is no common age relationship that can be applied generally to all toxicants. It is necessary to be aware that neo-natal and intact animals are not just small versions of the adult animals and that there is discontinuity if the surface area to bodyweight formulae are applied without regard to age, but by using the formula that uses the specified function constant k_s and varying that constant with age, a family of curves can be obtained that are similar to those for oxygen uptake (Zeuthen, 1953). However, Triggs and Nation (1975) have indicated that the extent of absorption alters little with age but that in old animals, protein binding, tissue distribution and renal, or other, clearance may be very different from those in the younger animal. For example, Smith and Rose (1977) have demonstrated that the apparent differences in the sensitivity of the lungs of rats to paraquat at different ages is directly related to plasma and lung concentrations of toxicant being affected by the renal clearance rates at different ages.

Sex

As a result of a survey of the acute oral and percutaneous toxicities of 98 pesticides to rats, Gaines (1969) concluded that when tested by the oral route the majority were more toxic to females than to males. Gaines found the reverse was true for only 9 of the 98 compounds tested; these exceptions were aldrin, chlordane, heptachlor, abate, imidan, methyl-parathion, fenchlorphos, schradan, and metepa.

Pallotta *et al.* (1962) investigated the toxicity of the antibiotic acetoxycycloheximide and found that the female rat and the female mouse were more susceptible than the corresponding males but that no sex difference was apparent when the compound was administered to dogs.

A review of the published literature on pesticides reveals that sex differences in response are common in rodents (Kato and Gillette, 1965) but much less common in other mammals, although the information on the latter is often not definitive. Even with rodents the pattern of sex differences is not always consistent, for example the organophosphorus insecticide mevinphos is more toxic to male Mongolian gerbils than to females (Maines and Westfall, 1971; Steen *et al.*, 1976) but the reverse is the case for rats (Gaines, 1960). These observations are in accord with published data on the metabolic activity for each species as measured by hexobarbitone sleeping time (Table 3.11).

Investigating the microsomal metabolism of some compounds *in vitro*, Kato and Gillette (1965) were able to demonstrate sex differences with rat liver preparations and they also found that the differences were inconsistent and depended on the substrates used. Comparable detailed studies have been reported by El Masry and Mannering (1974), El Masry *et al.* (1974), Cohen and Mannering (1974), and Sladek *et al.* (1974) all investigating the influence of sex on the response of rats to drugs. Kato and Onoda (1966) and Kato *et al.* (1971) studies the influence of morphine on microsomal drug-metabolizing agents and found that there were marked effects attributable to sex in rats but no such sex-related effects were found when they investigated guinea-pigs, rabbits, and mice.

By utilizing hepatic tissue from some mammalian species, Whitehouse and Ecobichon (1975) studies the formation of paraoxon from parathion and its subsequent hydrolysis; they found that only guinea-pigs and rats exhibited sex differences in activation (i.e. the males showed higher desulphurating ability than the females) and only in rats was a sex

Table 3.11 Relative hexobarbitone sleeping times for different rodent species of each sex

Sex	Mean sleeping time (min)		
	Mongolian gerbil[a]	Rat[b]*	Mouse[c]
Male	105 ± 9.6	22 ± 4	34 ± 5
Female	70 ± 6.9	67 ± 15	31 ± 5

[a]Data from Maines and Westfall (1971).
[b]Data from Quinn *et al.* (1958).
[c]Data from Vessell (1968).
*The reported sex difference does not occur in rats aged less than 4 weeks.

difference recorded for paraoxon hydrolysis (i.e. the males exhibited higher arylesterase activity than the females).

The nutritional status of animals can affect the acute response to toxic chemicals (Boyd *et al.*, 1970; Boyd, 1972). Within the controlled conditions of the laboratory even the response of fish to toxicants has been shown to be influenced by diet; Mehrle *et al.* (1973) fed rainbow trout on a range of commercially available fish foods and found that the piscicidal effect of chlordane, measured as LC_{50} (96 hours), varied between 9.2 µg/l (95% Confidence Limits 6.1–11.0 µg/l) and 47.0 µg/l (95% Confidence Limits 37.7–58.5 µg/l).

Similarly, the nutritional status of the animals used to prepare the tissues for *in vitro* studies can alter the whole quantitative pattern of microsomal metabolism and the amount of change may not always be the same for both sexes (Kato and Gillette, 1965). This finding might have important implications in *in vivo* acute toxicity tests since such tests are frequently carried out in animals following a period of restricted food intake.

Krasovskij (1975) studied data on the acute toxicities of 149 compounds and compared the results for males and females. He concluded that females tend to be more sensitive than males but that on average the differences are species-dependent and small. By arbitrarily defining the sensitivity of males as 1, the ratios for the 149 test products in females were:

Rat   0.88 ± 0.036

Mouse 0.92 ± 0.058

In this series of data, Krasovskij found very large sex differences only with organophosphates, parathion and disulfoton being three to eight times more toxic to females. Krasovskij found that some organophosphates were more toxic to males than to females, these included malathion, methylparathion, and fenchlorphos. The data of Gaines (1960) agree with this sex relationship but in the case of malathion Gaines found female rats more sensitive to acute intoxication than male rats.

Since cholinesterases are common target enzymes for many pesticides, it is relevant to consider the possibility of sex differences in relation to these enzymes. Shanor *et al.* (1961) found with humans that there is a statistically significant difference between the plasma cholinesterase activities of young healthy males and females (i.e. female plasma enzyme activity equivalent to between 64 and 74% of the male enzyme activity), but that this difference disappeared in older populations, the overall activity diminishing. These same investigators found no statistically different variation in the erythrocyte cholinesterase activity between males and females at any age. Naik *et al.* (1970) found that there was no significant difference in total brain cholinesterase activity or in total brain acetylcholine between male and female rats whereas Eben and Pilz (1967) found that the plasma cholinesterase of adult female rats exceeded that of the male rat by about threefold, although they found no significant difference in the erythrocyte cholinesterase activities between sexes. Although these reported investigations have been carried out in a comparative manner with respect to sex, some of the technical problems in investigating plasma, erythrocyte, and brain cholinesterases in different species have been demonstrated by Pickering and Pickering (1971, 1974, and 1977). Since choline, acetylcholine, and the cholinesterases are not uniformly distributed in the central nervous system (Stavinhova *et al.*, 1974) it may be deduced *a priori* that the distribution characteristics of a toxicant affecting these must be critical to its toxicity and this distribution characteristic may well be affected by the sex of the animal.

Working with the organophosphorus insecticide parathion, DuBois *et al.* (1949) showed that administration of diethylstilboestrol to male rats and testosterone to female rats could almost abolish the sex difference in response to acute intoxication by the pesticide. Robinson *et al.* (1978) found that premedication of rats with ethylestrenol gave some protection against intoxication with cholinesterase inhibitors.

Bedford and Hutson (1976) demonstrated that the excretion and distribution patterns for endrin and dieldrin are different in male and female rats. But in an earlier publication, Bedford *et al.* (1975) reported a much smaller sex difference between the acute LD_{50} values for endrin than has been reported by some other investigators (Treon *et al.*, 1955; Gaines, 1960).

The influence of sex on the toxicity of compounds has been the subject of review articles by Hathway (1970), Moore (1972), and Kato (1974).

Strain

Populations of animals may change their sensitivity to intoxication by chemicals (Meier, 1963a and 1963b; Guthrie *et al.*, 1971). These changes have proved to be a serious problem in pest control as well as in the laboratory. For example some wild rats have developed resistance to anticoagulant rodenticides (Gratz, 1973; Zimmermann and Matschiner, 1974).

Although strain-related responses (Hilado and Furst, 1978) and pharmacogenetics have been the subject of numerous reviews (Kalow, 1962 and 1965; Meier, 1963a and 1963b; Vessell, 1969; Hathway, 1970; Moore, 1972; Lang and Vessell, 1976), few investigators have studied mechanisms of variation in vertebrate animals (Becker, 1962) although exceptions are the studies on the sensitivity of rats to oxygen (Robinson *et al.*, 1967), to nitrous oxide (Green, 1968), and to warfarin (Davis and Davies, 1970; Zimmermann and Matschiner, 1974). Weaver and Kerley (1962) studied the responses of various strains of mice to *d*-amphetamine and Brown (1961) reported on the sleeping time responses of random bred, inbred, and F_1 hybrid mice to pentobarbitone sodium; later the same author (Brown, A. M., 1964 and 1965) also investigated the responses of different mouse strains to insulin. Hill *et al.* (1975) reported that the lethal dose of chloroform was four times higher to C57BL/6J mice than to male DBA/2J mice and that twice as much chloroform accumulated in the kidneys of the sensitive than in the kidneys of the resistant strains of mouse.

Miura *et al.* (1974) studied the acute toxicity of one batch of the pesticide technical BHC in five different strains of mice and found a wide range of sensitivities:

Strain	LD_{50} (no limits quoted) (mg/kg)
SS	411
CF No. 1	500
AA	802
C57BL/6	1 414
C3H/He	1 459

Haley *et al.* (1973) demonstrated a similar range of strain differences for mice in response to acute intoxication by *N*-2-fluorenylacetamide, a compound once developed as an insecticide.

Quinn *et al.* (1958) found strain differences when they investigated the metabolism of hexobarbitone, amidopyrine, antipyrine, and aniline.

Endrin resistance has been found to occur in wild pine mice (Webb and Horsfall, 1967) and this phenomenon has been studied in laboratory housed pine mice (*Mus pitymys pinetorum*) by Webb *et al.* (1973) and Petrella *et al.* (1975); the LD_{50} values obtained for endrin by these investigators ranged between 1.37 and 36.4 mg/kg.

Bedford and Hutson (1976) found that the faecal excretion of dieldrin was quantitatively different in LACG mice and CF No. 1 mice, 24 and 46% of the administered dose respectively.

The veterinary anthelmintic haloxon and some related di-(2-chloroethyl) aryl phosphates are known to cause ataxia in some sheep and not in others. This has been shown to be a genetic effect due to the presence or absence of a dominant allele in the different breeds of sheep (Lee, 1964).

It is pertinent to note that the growth and development characteristics for a species are, in part, a function of heredity (Goodrick, 1973), for these factors may influence sensitivity to toxicants. The shortfall in the understanding of pharmacogenetics in relation to the toxicity of pesticides has been acknowledged by the World Health Organization (Wld. Hlth. Org. Rep. Ser. No. 524, 1973).

Stress factors and rhythmic behaviour

Physiological rhythms are complex interactions of bodily response to time-spaced extraneous factors (Winfree, 1975). Martinez-O'Ferrall (1968) stated that the habitat of life exhibits a recurrence of a sequence of events in an orderly manner vectorially related to time. Intervention of a toxic response must interfere with the normal rhythmic patterns and biological cybernetics; however, there is very little evidence of serious differences in acute toxicity being manifested by time rhythms (Scheving et al., 1974). The factors that influence the frequency and synchronization of the biological functions are called 'zeitgeber' and these may be numerous and also interactive.

Circadian differences in response to various unrelated chemicals such as nikethamide (Carlsson and Serin, 1950a and 1950b), ethanol (Haus and Halberg, 1959), librium (Marte and Halberg, 1961), methopyrapone (Ertel et al., 1964), and ouabain (Nelson et al., 1971) have been observed in the mouse. Indeed, Halberg et al. (1960) demonstrated that there would be a potency ratio variation of from 3.2 to 1 for the bioassay of Escherichia coli endotoxin carried out at time intervals of 12 hours. Working with rats, Lenox and Frazier (1972) demonstrated that mortality due to methadone could be influenced by the circadian cycle. On a more coarse time-scale, Weinstock and Shoham (1974) demonstrated seasonal variation in the sensitivity of guinea-pig tissues and agonists.

Measurements of metabolic activity of liver homogenates from rats were found to correlate both with periods of light and dark exposure of the animals and also with the plasma corticosterone concentrations (Jori et al., 1971). This work was extended by Holcslaw et al. (1975) who showed that total light exposure or reversal of the light–dark cycles altered the response accordingly.

Stress has been defined as the reactions of the animal body to forces of a deleterious nature, infections, and various abnormal states that tend to disturb the normal physiological rhythms and equilibrium. Thus there are clear relationships between biorhythms, stress, and endocrine function (Martinez-O'Ferrall, 1968; Bunning, 1967). It has been demonstrated that injections of adrenocorticotrophic hormone (Vaccarezza and Willson, 1964a and 1964b) caused increases both in plasma and cell cholinesterases in rats, but the same investigators found that adrenalectomy caused a progressive fall in the circulating cell cholinesterase but had no effect on the plasma cholinesterase in rats (Vaccarezza and Willson, 1965). In man, injections of adrenocorticotrophic hormone also gave rise to increases in plasma and circulating cell cholinesterases (Vaccarezza and Peltz, 1960). Naik et al. (1970) studied two forms of stress on rat brain acetylcholine and cholinesterases and found that with the physical stress of vertical spinning there was an immediate and significant fall in brain acetylcholine and a rise in cholinesterase activity, but that stress induced by fasting caused the reverse effect with both variables.

Stockinger (1953) has indicated the considerable effect that stress can have on the dose distribution of some chemical elements in the body.

Investigating the organophosphorus insecticide parathion in rats, Kling and Long (1969) demonstrated that dietary stress could influence the time course of the cell cholinesterase response but had little effect on the quantitative response. Murphy (1969a) found that exposure of rats to some organophosphates resulted in increased concentrations of plasma corticosterone and that inhibition of liver metabolism of steroid hormones can also occur, this latter observation agrees with the findings of Conney *et al.*, (1967).

The insecticide 2,2-bis(*p*-chlorophenyl)-1:1-dichloroethane (DDD) has been shown to cause adrenocortical ablation in the dog (Küchmeister *et al.*, 1955).

Stress due to fasting has been shown to alter the permeability of the blood–brain barrier to some chemicals (Angel, 1969). Selective starvation can also influence sensitivity to toxicants; Boyd *et al.* (1970) demonstrated that feeding protein-deficient or protein-rich diets to rats could profoundly alter the LD_{50} values for many pesticides (Table 3.12).

With some toxicants the influence of either multiple or single housing of the experimental animals can significantly alter the results of toxicity tests (Chance, 1947; Chance and Mackintosh, 1962).

When considering stress factors and rhythms it is essential not to overlook social and other ambient factors (Lang and Vessell, 1976). With experimental populations the influence of caging or housing can be a major influence, particularly with gregarious animals such as rodents (Chance, 1947; Chance and Mackintosh, 1962; Davis, 1962; Wiberg and Grice, 1965; Baer, 1971). Hibernating animals may respond to toxicants differently during the dormant stage that when active, this has been demonstrated by Scaife and Campbell (1958), who demonstrated that the anticholinesterase agent *O,O*-diethyl-*S*-2-diethylaminoethyl phosphonothiolate it significantly more toxic when injected intraperitoneally into

Table 3.12   The influence of dietary protein on the acute toxicities of several pesticides to rats (Data from Boyd *et al.*, 1970)

	Relative LD_{50} values				
	Protein (%, w) in diet*				
	0	3.5	9.0	26.0†	81.0
Captan	2 100.0	26.3	1.2	1.0	2.4
Carbaryl	8.6	6.5	1.1	1.0	1.0
Chlorpropam	8.7	4.0	1.7	1.0	—
Diazinon	7.4	1.9	1.8	1.0	2.0
DDT	4.0	2.9	1.5	1.0	2.0
Endosulphan	20.0	4.3	1.8	1.0	1.0
Lindane	12.3	1.9	1.0	1.0	1.8
Monuron	11.5	3.0	1.8	1.0	—

*Amount of protein fed to the rats for 28 days after weaning.
†Normal amount of protein fed to rats—value for relative LD_{50}'s taken as 1.0.

hibernating hamsters than when injected into active hamsters. During sleep, absorption of toxicants from the gastro-intestinal tract is sometimes diminished (Mattock and McGilveray, 1973).

In a series of experiments carried out over a period of 500 days from December 1960 to April 1962, Selisko et al. (1963) found that there was no correlation between response and light, nor was there any correlation with season, following intraperitoneal injection of aqueous solutions of nicotine bitartrate into rats. However, these workers did find a correlation between response and ambient humidity.

Stress due to infection can alter the response of animals to toxicants. Safarov and Aleskerov (1972) found that the dipping of sheep in an ectoparasiticide depressed antibody production and that sleep convalescing from infections died. The hepatitis virus in ducks has been shown to influence hepatic microsomal enzyme activity and this can increase the LD_{50} values of pesticides such as dieldrin and DDT in ducks (Friend and Trainer, 1972). It has been suggested that some pesticides may adversely affect natural immunological defence systems, although this is associated more with persistent pesticides retained in the animals (Wasserman et al., 1969).

Temperature

In the context of toxicology, temperature must include both the ambient temperature and the physiological thermoregulation of the animals. The ambient temperature is closely associated with ambient humidity and the two variables are conveniently considered together (Lang and Vessell, 1976).

The relevant investigations of Krebs (1950) and Zeuthen (1953) in relation to oxygen uptake, tissue heat, and ontogenetic recapitulation have been referred to earlier in this chapter. Belehrádek (1957) consolidated many years' of his own and other investigators' research and produced a unified theory of cellular rate processes based on an analysis of temperature action; he concluded that the rate of biological processes is primarily determined by protoplasmic resistance opposing free movement of molecules travelling within living matter rather than the rate of chemical change considered by itself. Belehrádek (1957) was enthusiastic about the relationship of Slotte's temperature–viscosity relationship formula to the cellular system and he further related these relationships to the Van't Hoff–Arrhenius temperature coefficients; however, the shortcomings of the latter coefficients in vertebrate animals have been reviewed by Brody (1964).

Usinger (1957) observed that drug responses in animals were sometimes paradoxically affected by the ambient temperature. He investigated this phenomenon in mice and found with that species the mean oxygen consumption for unit bodyweight in unit time diminishes when the temperature increases from 25 to 30 °C, then rises again when the ambient temperature is 35 °C (i.e. the minimum oxygen utilization is at 30 °C). However, Usinger (1957) also measured the rectal temperature of the mice and found that the minimum rectal temperature occurred when the ambient temperature was 25 °C, either side of this value the rectal temperature was higher. Ahdaya et al. (1976) investigated themoregulation in mice exposed to parathion, carbaryl, and DDT; their studies were carried out at 1, 27, and 38 °C and each of the three pesticides was found to be least toxic at 27 °C (Table 3.13). Many drugs can profoundly affect the body temperature (Cremer and Bligh, 1969) and ambient temperature can affect response to many drugs (Doull, 1972); the same applies to several types of pesticides. Doull (1972) presented the hypothesis that temperature is directly correlated with the magnitude and inversely correlated with the duration of drug response in biological systems; however, it is clear that the effect of temperature on one variable may not necessarily be predictive for effects on other pharmacological responses.

Atabaev and Kur (1978) investigated the effects of pesticides on energy metabolism under conditions of elevated temperature and found that several organophosphate and carbamate anticholinesterase agents exhibited less effect on cholinesterases, in vivo, at high temperatures.

Investigating the toxicity of parathion to mice at various temperatures, Baetjer and Smith (1956) found that the onset of death, the rate of dying and the rate of recovery were more rapid, the survival time for fatal cases was shorter, and the mortality was higher at 35.6 °C than at 22.8 °C; at 15.6 °C the onset of death was delayed and the final, but not the early, mortality exceeded that at 22.8°C. Baetjer and Smith (1956) went on to investigate the influence of pre-exposure and post-exposure temperatures on the response of mice and found that mortality varied directly with pre- and inversely with post-exposure ambient temperatures. These workers concluded that their results could not be attributed to acceleration of chemical reactions in vivo but were due to changes in the rates of absorption and other physical factors. Keplinger et al. (1959) followed up this study with an investigation of 58 compounds and their acute toxicity to

Table 3.13 The influence of ambient temperature on the acute intraperitoneal toxicity of three pesticides to mice (Data from Ahdaya et al., 1976)

	LD_{50} values (mg/kg) (95% confidence limits)		
	Temperature		
	1 °C	27 °C	38 °C
Parathion	16.5 (13.2–20.6)	29 (23–35.9)	11.3 (8.3–15.2)
Carbaryl	263 (173–400)	588 (420–822)	112 (66–191)
DDT	750 (535–1 050)	1175 (758–1 821)	875 (565–1 385)

rats under different ambient conditions. Among the compounds investigated by Keplinger *et al.* were the pesticides warfarin, DNOC, pentachlorophenol, DDT, and strychnine with the following general findings: to rats, warfarin was less toxic at 26 °C than at 8 °C or 36 °C, DNOC and pentachlorophenol were less toxic at 8 °C than at 26 °C and less toxic at 26 °C than at 36 °C; DDT was equi-toxic at 8 °C and 26 °C, but much more toxic at 36 °C; strychnine was equi-toxic at 8 °C and 36 °C but less toxic at 26 °C.

A large variation in the sensitivity of rats to acute intoxication by the rodenticide alphanaphthylthiourea (ANTU) at different temperatures was reported by Meyer and Karel (1948), and it was found that the response was not linear (Table 3.14).

The influence of the pesticide dinitro-*o*-cresol (DNOC) has been well documented in relation to body and ambient temperatures (Wolfe *et al.*, 1961). Hayes (1963) pointed out that DNOC is more effective in raising body temperature in humans if the ambient temperature is 22 °C or over; if the ambient temperature is 16 °C or less, increased oxidation and pyrexia are not produced and, indeed, the converse may apply (i.e. oxidation is reduced and body cooling may occur). Ambient temperature has been shown to be critical in the response of rodents and birds to the rodenticide and avicide alphachloralose (Cornwell, 1969; Cornwell and Bull, 1967), when the thermoregulatory mechanisms within the Class Aves are considered (King and Farner, 1961) the importance of ambient temperature on the response of birds to pesticides becomes apparent (Brown, V. K. H., 1974).

With organophosphates, there has long been concern about the influence of ambient working conditions on toxicity (Quinby and Lemmon, 1958). By measuring the urinary output of *p*-nitrophenol. Funckes *et al.* (1963) showed that the rate of absorption of parathion in man was temperature-related and that the excretion of *p*-nitrophenol varied directly with temperature over the range 14.4–40.5 °C. Durham *et al.* (1972) considered that in field use the temperature effect is likely to be most apparent in terms of percutaneous rather than inhalational exposure; however, Grigorowa and Binnewies (1973) and Gohlke and Grigorowa (1973) have demonstrated, using rats, that temperature can profoundly affect the

Table 3.14 The relationship between ambient temperature and LD_{50} for ANTU administered to rats. (Data from Meyer and Karel, 1948)

Temperature (°F)	LD_{50} (mg/kg) $\pm$ S.E.
36–38	1.90 ± 0.13
46–50	2.91 ± 0.24
68–75	4.03 ± 0.34
87–90	1.23 ± 0.23

inhalation toxicity of tinox, dimethoate and methylparathion. Caution is the interpretation of results with rats treated with organophosphates is always essential as it is easy to cause sensitivity to ambient temperature change by inducing hypothermia in the animals at the same time that the cholinesterase is depressed; this effect was reported by Meeter and Wolthius (1968).

White *et al.* (1976) demonstrated that there is a negative temperature coefficient in the response of female rats to intoxication by the insecticide cismethrin when it is administered by mouth but not when it is injected intravenously (Table 3.15).

Investigators at Forschungsinstitut für Bioklimatologie, Berlin (Selisko *et al.*, 1963), investigated the effects of various exogenous factors on the acute intraperitoneal toxicity of nicotine to mice and decided that the only factor that caused a significant effect was air humidity. In general this would have been less surprising if ambient humidity had a more marked effect on absorption through the skin (Neely *et al.*, 1967), however the influence of humidity might be difficult to predict since the relationship between transepidermal water loss in sweating animals and the ambient humidity is not linear (Grice *et al.*, 1972) and the situation is even more complicated in the non-sweating species (Neely *et al.*, 1967).

The state of physiological hydration of the test animal can be very important in influencing the toxic response. Investigating two toxicants, caffeine and dextroamphetamine, Muller and Vernikos-Danellis (1968) demonstrated that the LD_{50} values in mice were profoundly influenced by ambient temperature and that physiological dehydration of the animals produced a marked potentiation of the toxicity of caffeine at 30 °C whereas the effect on dextroamphetamine was much less; there was some increase in toxicity at 22 °C with both compounds but at 15 °C there was no effect on the LD_{50} for dextroamphetamine and only a very small effect on the value for caffeine.

The influence of temperature on the sensitivity of poikilothermal animals to toxicants is subject to much variation (Holden, 1973). This sensitivity variation is dependent on the species and on the pesticide and may be

Table 3.15   The relationship between ambient temperature and LD_{50} for cismethrin administered by different routes. (Data from White *et al.*, 1976)

Route	Temperature (°C)	LD_{50} (mg/kg) (95% confidence limits)	
Oral	3–4	157	(125–197)
Oral	19–21	197	(139–280)
Oral	29–31	>1 000	
I.V.	19–21	4.5	(3.5–5.6)
I.V.	29–31	4.5	(3.5–5.6)

manifested by an increase or a decrease with increase in temperature, this has been demonstrated with endrin (Macek *et al.*, 1969) and DDT (Cope, 1964). Lakota (1974) determined the LC_{50} values for a large number of pesticides at 96 hours exposure using a species of carp and a species of trout; he found that in the majority of cases the toxicity was significantly greater at elevated temperatures, his exceptions were the herbicide 2,4-D and the insecticide DDT, these two exhibited a decreased toxicity. Pyrethrum extract and some pyrethroids were found to be more toxic to fish at 12 °C than at 22 °C but Mauck and Olson (1976) found that the reverse was true for *d-trans*-allethrin.

CHAPTER 4

Dose and dosage

The term 'dose' is defined as the quantity of toxicant administered to, or received by, the animal at one time or in a given period of time. 'Dosage' refers to the administration of a toxicant in doses.

Conventionally, dosage information in acute toxicity is expressed in abbreviated form to relate the amount of toxicant to some physical property of the exposed animal. For example, the LD_{50} value for a toxicant may be expressed in milligrams of toxicant per kilogram bodyweight of animal and this is generally written in the form mg/kg or, to be in line with the physical sciences and engineering, mg kg^{-1}. Although the quantity of toxicant may be expressed in any of several different units (e.g. mg, mol, ml, etc.) it is unusual for bodyweight to be expressed in units other than the kilogram even if the species is small or large.

The ultimate response (Chapter 2) as a result of acute exposure is dependent on the amount of toxicant at the critical target sites. The amount of toxicant at the target site is dependent, in part, on the dose. Between exposure to the dose and the response there are four major occurrences. The first three occurrences are absorption, metabolism, and excretion (Scheme 4.1) and in this context metabolism includes both detoxification and toxification processes. Theoretical relationships can be identified to explain the processes involved (Janku and Farghalli, 1971; Prescott, 1972; Piotrowski, 1972; Janku, 1973; Natoff, 1973). The fourth occurrence, distribution within the body, is critical to the toxicology of chemicals. Examples of the importance of distribution include the physical properties that are essential for penetration of the blood–brain barrier, such that the toxicant may reach targets in the brain (Rall, 1971; Oldendorf, 1974), and the ability for uptake of some toxicants by the body fat, which comprises about 20% of the total body mass, and the subsequent release to produce toxic manifestations (Mark, 1971; Davies et al., 1975).

In addition to the above, response has been shown to be a function of route of exposure (Chapters 2 and 5) and also species exposed (Chapter 3). Some of the more important remaining factors are:

THE BODY-DOSE-EFFECT RELATIONSHIP

The expression of acute toxicity in terms of amount of toxicant per unit of bodyweight has become an almost universal convention. Thus there is an implication that the physiological capacity of a whole animal remains constant throughout its life and this is clearly a fallacious assumption

Scheme 4.1

Simple formalized presentation of the hypothesis that it is not the fact of absorption that kills but rather the rate of absorption (Brown, 1968).

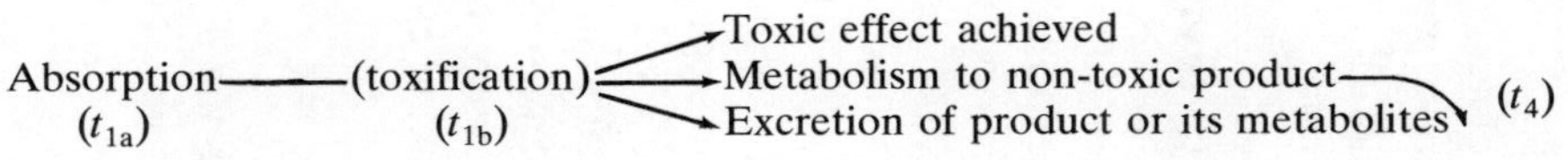

$$\text{Absorption} \xrightarrow[\;(t_{1a})\;]{\;\text{(toxification)}\;(t_{1b})} \begin{array}{l} \text{Toxic effect achieved} \\ \text{Metabolism to non-toxic product} \xrightarrow{\;\;\;\;\;} (t_4) \\ \text{Excretion of product or its metabolites} \end{array}$$

t_1, t_2 etc. = relative rates.

If $[(t_{1a}) + (t_{1b})]$ is rapid, then the probability of $(t_2) \geqslant [(t_3) + (t_4) + (t_5)]$ is achieved.

But if $[(t_{1a}) + (t_{1b})]$ is slow, then the probability of $(t_2) \leqslant [(t_3) + (t_4) + (t_5)]$ is achieved.

Should toxification not be necessary, then (t_{1b}) is negligible; however, where toxification is essential (e.g. parathion $\rightarrow$ paraoxon) the relationship between (t_{1a}) and (t_{1b}) is very important.

70

(Holliday *et al.*, 1967) and, since there are large differences between the basal metabolisms of different species that may be correlated with the surface area of the body, body surface-area might be considered to be a better alternative to the bodyweight for the expression of dosage (Freireich *et al.*, 1966; Mellett, 1969).

Rall and North (1953), Angelakos (1960), and Pallotta *et al.* (1962) have published examples of the artefacts that can occur when dosage is expressed in terms of unit bodyweight and they set out to show that the expression in terms of dose per whole animal is more meaningful.

Stockinger (1953) reported that dosage can profoundly influence the pattern of distribution of some chemical elements in the body. The mechanisms involved in the distribution were the existence of colloidal phagocytosable cations, the occurrence of metal–protein complexing and other physiological regulatory mechanisms.

CONCENTRATION–TIME OF EXPOSURE RELATIONSHIPS

Bliss (1940) stated that a time factor may be involved, not only as a stimulus such that the length of exposure to a given concentration determines the amount fixed within the organism, but also as the measured response to a given dose of toxicant which may or may not involve a time factor in its administration. In acute toxicity, the time of exposure is generally considered as that period during which the animal is exposed to the toxicant from extracorporeal sources although acute manifestations due to the release of toxicants from intracorporeal sources (e.g. release from depots in the body fat) must not be wholly discounted (Janku *et al.*, 1971).

Throughout this book acute exposure has been defined as being an exposure on one occasion only or, exceptionally, multiple exposures within a time limit of 24 hours. However, a more closely specified time limit for exposure is required for two types of acute exposure.

(i) Environmental exposure

This type of exposure is generally limited to inhalation toxicity or the toxicity of chemicals to aquatic animals. Two distinct situations can be attained:

(a) Static

There is an initial concentration of toxicant in the environment and this concentration diminishes because of uptake by the animal, adsorption on to surfaces, degradation etc. and there is no source of replenishment of the toxicant in the environment.

(b) Dynamic

The concentration of toxicant in the environment undergoes a process of replenishment offsetting any physical removal of the toxicant that may be occurring.

Environmental exposures are not generally expressed in terms of dosage but rather the term concentration to produce the defined toxic response is used, time of exposure being an essential variable. Thus the concentration of a vapour that would kill 50% of a population of animals in 8 hours is expressed as the LC_{50} value, 8 hours (see Chapter 2).

The results of tests involving the three variables concentration, time, and response can be analysed mathematically (Box, 1954) or they can be expressed in terms of three-dimensional graphs (Skidmore, 1974). A less detailed method of analysis involves using multiple graphs in which two of the three variables only are analysed on each graph (Tammes et al., 1967), for example using concentration and response as variables with time arbitrarily fixed.

Some investigators advocate studies with specified concentrations of toxicant in the environment and the use of time and response as variables (Zaeva et al., 1968) but others suggest the use of constant time intervals in order to produce an integrated time–effect curve (Brittain and Spencer, 1965). Sometimes it is found that there is an approximate relationship, that the product of concentration and time to produce a defined response is constant (Haber, 1924), but this approximation is not wholly true (MacFarland, 1975) and should be used cautiously.

Jenkins et al. (1976) found that survival time data for mixtures of toxicants can be modelled on the equation:

$$C = C_0 + \left[\frac{\beta}{(MST - T_0)} \right]$$

when,

C = concentration of A in mixture of A and B

C_0 = estimate of the asymptote of concentration of A as survival time increases towards infinity

β = slope of the curve of concentration versus the reciprocal of the survival time

MST = mean survival time for a group of experimental animals in which all died during the exposure

T_0 = an estimate of the asymptote of the mean survival time approached as concentration of component A increases towards infinity.

THE INFLUENCE OF FORMULATION ON TOXIC EFFECTS

The efficacy and efficiency of pesticides are very dependent on their presentation to the target pest. The acute toxicity of any pesticide to non-target species is also dependent on the form of its presentation (Hayes

Table 4.1 The acute toxicity of diquat to fathead minnows.
(Data from Calderbank, 1968)

Water hardness in mg/l $CaCO_3$	LC_{50} mg/l of diquat		
	24 hours	48 hours	96 hours
320–382 ('hard')	756	220	130
19–27 ('soft')	140	22	12

and Pearce, 1953; Freed and Witt, 1969; Done and Peart, 1971; Staiff *et al.*, 1973) and the duration of exposure (Brown and Muir, 1971). Both of these influences can be illustrated by reference to some examples of the acute toxicity of pesticides to fish. Hughes and Davis (1963), investigating the toxicology of the herbicide 2,4-dichlorophenoxyacetic acid (2,4-D), found that formulated as the alkanolamine salt the 24 hour LC_{50} value to bluegills (*Lepomis macrochirus*) was greater than 450 mg/l acid equivalent but when the isopropyl ester of 2,4-D was used the comparable LC_{50} value was found to be less than 1 mg/l acid equivalent. Calderbank (1968) investigated the toxicology of the bipyridylium herbicide diquat using fathead minnows (*Pimephales promelas*) and found that water hardness profoundly affected the result but that duration of exposure was a critical factor (Table 4.1).

Water hardness has also been shown to affect the response by fish to intoxication by pyrethrum extracts and synthetic pyrethroids (Mauck and Olson, 1976).

THE INFLUENCE OF VEHICLE ON ACUTE TOXICITY

The word 'vehicle' is a general term used to describe those constituents of pesticide formulations other than the major active components and may include solvents, carriers, surfactants etc. The formulation of a pesticide can profoundly affect both its efficacy against the pest and its acute toxicity to non-target species. Formulation may either increase or diminish the acute toxicity properties of a chemical or even, on occasions, not significantly affect the acute toxicity either way, and these influences may be brought about by one or more of the following mechanisms:

(i) Effect on rate of absorption

Whatever the route of exposure the vehicle can influence absorption but there is no single relationship between either the quantitative or the qualitative effect on different routes of uptake. The intrinsic absorption characteristics of all chemicals are rooted in their physico-chemical properties (Ferguson, 1939; Brodie and Hogben, 1957; Schanker, 1960; Barr, 1969; Idson, 1971) and formulations of pesticides should be designed to accentuate the physical properties that are desirable for maximal efficacy and to minimize those properties that are undesirable such as the toxicity to non-target species.

The vehicle may be chosen to have an effect on the physiology of the target species, for example, the vehicle may aid the penetration of an insecticide through the insect cuticle. The influence of the same vehicle may be similar on the skin of non-target species and as a consequence the uptake of the pesticide by exposed non-target species may be increased, thus increasing the hazard factors. The effect of a vehicle at the absorptive site in the non-target species may be only functional or, in some cases, actual morphological change may also be apparent (Winne, 1970; Scheuplein and Ross, 1970).

(ii) Effect on bioavailability of the toxicant

Bioavailability changes may be brought about by changes in the physico-chemical properties of the toxicant in relation to the physiological milieu. In the case of solids an increase or a decrease in particle size can markedly alter the absorption characteristics from the respiratory tract (Morrow, 1960) and from the alimentary tract (Malone, 1964; Fincher, 1968; Wolter et al., 1972); even in those cases where a pesticide can be absorbed through the skin from the solid state, for example dieldrin (Negherbon, 1959; Bojanowska and Brzezicka-Bak, 1967), the particle size may be critical to the response.

Other physical factors influencing bioavailability of toxicant from pesticide formulations include the viscosity of suspensions (Ritschel et al., 1974) and the presence of materials that influence surface tension (Eickholt and White, 1960).

Sometimes toxicity is influenced by the intentional or unintentional interactions of the toxicant with formulation components. Some pesticides are insoluble in most vehicles but liquid formulations are prepared by interactive complexing or solubilization of the pesticide. For example, the herbicide 2,4-D is active as the parent acid (2,4-dichlorophenoxyacetic acid) but may be converted into various salts or esters to facilitate formulation (Way, 1969); these variants also affect the acute toxicity of the compounds to animals as well as to plants.

2,4-D
(2,4-Dichlorophenoxyacetic acid)

The toxic hazard can sometimes be reduced by adsorption of the pesticides on to inert fillers such as china clay. The same principle has been adapted for the therapeutic treatment of some types of pesticide intoxication and to achieve this, activated charcoal or kaolin is administered to absorb toxicants in the alimentary canal, thus diminishing absorption. Diminished absorption of toxicants from the alimentary canal by the administration of milk is also well known; Talanov and Leshchev (1972) investigated the influence of various vehicles, including milk, on the acute oral toxicity of the insecticide hexachlorocyclohexane (HCH) to mice and reported the approximate LD_{50} values shown in Table 4.2.

$$
\begin{array}{c}
HCl \\
ClHC \overset{C}{\diagdown} CHCl \\
ClH\overset{|}{C} \overset{|}{\diagdown}_{C} CHCl \\
HCl
\end{array}
$$

Hexachlorocyclohexane (gamma-BHC)

Chemical interactions between pesticide and vehicle can alter the toxicological properties of both components (Casida and Sanderson, 1963; Dowden and Bennett, 1965; Loen and Engstrom-Heg, 1970; Venezky, 1971). The types of changes are:

(iii) Synergistic, additive, and antagonistic interactions of toxicant and vehicle

Data obtained for the acute toxicity of a pesticide as a formulation are capable of the same mathematical interpretation as for any other mixture of toxicants (Plackett and Hewlett, 1948 and 1952). The toxicity of a pesticide may be increased or decreased by use of formulation techniques (Eickholt and White, 1960; Casida and Sanderson, 1963; Brown and Muir, 1971); in practice it is not always possible to obtain optimum efficacy of the pesticide and achieve minimum toxicity.

The concentration of toxicant in relation to the vehicle can be very important. Absorption may be facilitated or diminished by change in toxicant concentration and there is no single correlation between concentration

Table 4.2 The acute oral toxicity of technical hexachlorocyclohexane to mice. (Data from Talanov and Leshchev, 1972)

Vehicle	LD_{50} value in mg/kg of HCH
Vegetable oil	68
Aqueous emulsion	165
Aqueous polyglycol suspension	112
Egg albumen	118
Milk	364.5

and uptake, the relationship is dependent on the individual chemical involved and on the route of exposure (Ferguson, 1962; Crawford et al., 1965; Goodman and Gilman, 1970; Borowitz et al., 1971).

The influence of vehicle on acute toxicity may be dependent on the target species. For example, the acute oral toxicity of the acaricide tetrasul to rats was found by Verschuuren et al. (1973) to be slightly less when administered in arachis oil than when administered in olive oil, but administered to guinea-pigs the differential between the toxicities of the two solutions was far greater (Table 4.3).

Tetrasul

A practical problem for the experimental toxicologist is the formulation of candidate pesticides for the purpose of exposing experimental animals. For investigative purposes, pesticides that are liquid at room temperature can be administered undiluted and those solid pesticides that are water soluble may be administered to the animals as aqueous solutions. Undiluted solid pesticides can be administered in gelatine capsules to some test species but this technique is generally impractical with small species such as rodents. Ultimately, the pesticide under investigation must be tested in the formulation that is to be used for pest control but details of these formulations will not be available until the early investigations on the compounds have been carried out.

The idea of using the almost universal solvent dimethyl sulphoxide (DMSO) as a solvent for screening acute toxicity tests with new pesticides was developed (Brown et al., 1963). Later Weiss and Orzel (1967), while working at the U.S. Food and Drug Administration, published comparative data for the acute toxicity to rats of several pesticides formulated as solu-

Table 4.3 Acute oral LD_{50} values for the acaracide tetrasul administered to rats and guinea-pigs as solutions in olive oil and arachis oil. (Data from Verschuuren et al., 1973)

| Solvent | Sex | LD_{50} values (95% confidence limits) in g/kg | |
		Guinea-pig	Rat
Olive oil	Male	0.52 (0.25–1.10)	3.55 (2.72–4.63)
	Female	0.50 (0.23–1.10)	3.65 (2.67–4.98)
Arachis oil	Male	8.25 (3.97–17.1)	8.25 (3.97–17.1)
	Female	8.80 (5.22–14.8)	6.81 (3.96–11.7)

tions in DMSO, dimethyl formamide (DMF), dimethyl acetamide (DMA), propylene glycol, corn oil (containing 10% DMF as co-solvent), or as aqueous suspensions. Weiss and Orzel concluded that DMSO was the most satisfactory solvent for screening pesticides for acute toxicity by both the oral and the intraperitoneal routes. Other comparisons of the cute toxicity of pesticides dissolved in DMSO with that of pesticides dissolved in numerous other solvents have been reported by Worthley and Schott (1966) using mice and by Bartsch et al. (1976) in relation to both rats and mice; a detailed study of the acute toxicity of DMSO to several other species has been reported by Mason (1971) and Noel et al. (1975).

Although DMSO is very useful as a solvent for acute toxicity tests, caution is required as it is possible for chemical interactions to occur between the toxicant and the DMSO (Venezky, 1971). Although Ben et al. (1964) demonstrated little pharmacological interaction when several standard drugs were administered in DMSO solution. Kocsis et al. (1968) found that DMSO potentiated the acute toxicities of several hydrocarbon solvents and in a more complex situation Mancini and Kocsis (1974) found that DMSO increased the acute toxicity of carbon tetrachloride to rats but also diminished its hepatotoxicity; these investigators consider that the DMSO probably acted by free-radical scavenging in this interaction. Boyer (personal communication, 1972) found that DMSO could affect the acute toxicity of some organophosphorus compounds and reduce their acute toxicity rating (Table 4.4).

All vehicles exert some influence on the acute toxicity of the pesticide under investigation and, as with DMSO, the influence may be underesti-

$$C_2H_5O \quad O \quad CHCl$$

Chlorfenvinphos

Table 4.4 The acute oral toxicity of chlorfenvinphos to rats with and without exposure to dimethyl sulphoxide (DMSO)

Chlorfenvinphos dosed	Pre-exposure treatment of animals	LD$_{50}$ in mg/kg (95% confidence limits) of chlorfenvinphos
Aqueous suspension*	None	11 (8.5–14)
DMSO solution	None	33 (28–41)
Aqueous suspension*	DMSO 6 ml/kg, 30 min before exposure to chlorfenvinphos	80 (67–93)

*Contained 1% m/v carboxymethylcellulose as suspending agent.

mated by some investigators. Two examples of solvents that have been the subject of adverse comment are dimethyl formamide (Tanaka, 1971) and propylene glycol (Zaroslinski *et al.* (1971), both of these have been used by experimental toxicologists as solvents for use in acute toxicology testing.

Two solvents that may be used for oral administration of some pesticides with the advantage that they are suitable for intravenous toxicity testing as well are glycerol formal (Sanderson, 1959) and tetramethylurea (Dixon *et al.*, 1966). Glycerol formal is a mixture of two chemicals, 4-hydroxymethyl-1,3-dioxalane and 5-hydroxy-1,3-dioxane, and has been used in the investigation of the acute toxicology of pyrethrin and some synthetic pyrethroids (Verschoyle and Barnes, 1972). Tetramethylurea has an oral LD_{50} value between 2.5 and 3 g/kg to rats and mice whereas glycerol formal is even less toxic with an oral LD_{50} value in excess of 8 g/kg to both rats and mice.

The 2-alkoxy short chain derivatives of ethanol (alternatively known as glycol ethers) are solvents of increasing interest in pesticide formulations. Although ethanol, 2-methoxy ethanol, and 2-ethoxy ethanol are reasonably non-toxic, all three are more acutely toxic than DMSO when administered alone.

Hexylene glycol is widely used in commercial formulations of pesticides and has a low acute toxicity rating. Several other solvents have been investigated for acute toxicity to rats of three different age groups (i.e. 14 days old, young adults, and older adults) by Kimura *et al.* (1971); 8 of the 16 solvents investigated were more toxic to the 14 day old rats than to the young adults (defined by Kimura *et al.* as being in the weight range 80 to 160 g) but more surprisingly, 2 of the 16, cyclohexane and methanol, were more toxic to the older adults (defined as being in the weight range 300 to 470 g) than to the young adults.

For experimental toxicology, vegetable oils such as corn oil, olive oil, and peanut oil are often used (Treon *et al.*, 1955; Gaines, 1960 and 1969; Verschuuren *et al.*, 1973). Emulsions have entirely different characteristics as solvents for lipophilic chemicals than either oil or water alone (Talanov and Leshechev, 1972).

Gaines (1960) described acute toxicity data for the carbamate insecticide 1-isopropyl-3-methyl-5-pyrazolyl dimethylcarbamate (ISOLAN)[a] to rats. Gaines concluded that this compound was more toxic by the percutaneous route than when administered orally. It is apparent that, given a suitable solvent common to both routes of exposure, this carbamate is not really more toxic by the skin route than when administered orally (Brown, 1968) and even if the toxicity data are extrapolated by regression analysis there is no lethal dose value at which the compound is more toxic by the percutaneous route than when administered orally.

A presentation of the influences of formulation on the acute toxicity of pesticides is given in Scheme 4.2.

[a]ISOLAN is a registered trade-mark of Ciba-Geigy AG.

Scheme 4.2

Formalized presentation of the possible influences of formulation on the acute toxicity of a pesticide

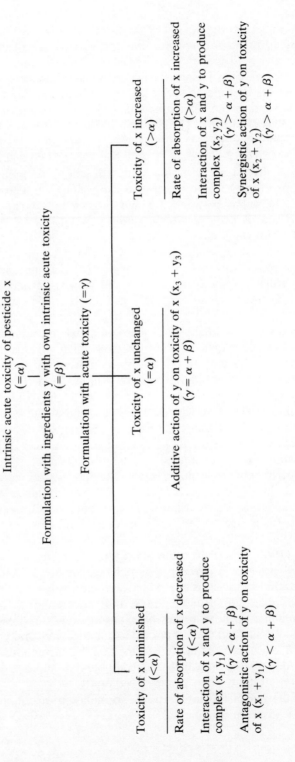

Intrinsic acute toxicity of pesticide x
$(=\alpha)$

Formulation with ingredients y with own intrinsic acute toxicity
$(=\beta)$

Formulation with acute toxicity $(=\gamma)$

Toxicity of x diminished
$(<\alpha)$

Rate of absorption of x decreased
$(<\alpha)$
Interaction of x and y to produce complex $(x_1 y_1)$
$(\gamma < \alpha + \beta)$
Antagonistic action of y on toxicity of x $(x_1 + y_1)$
$(\gamma < \alpha + \beta)$

Toxicity of x unchanged
$(=\alpha)$

Additive action of y on toxicity of x $(x_3 + y_3)$
$(\gamma = \alpha + \beta)$

Toxicity of x increased
$(>\alpha)$

Rate of absorption of x increased
$(>\alpha)$
Interaction of x and y to produce complex $(x_2 y_2)$
$(\gamma > \alpha + \beta)$
Synergistic action of y on toxicity of x $(x_2 + y_2)$
$(\gamma > \alpha + \beta)$

THE INFLUENCE OF MULTIPLE EXPOSURE

The responses associated with acute exposure to a pesticide may be modified by previous sub-lethal exposure of the animal to the same toxicant or by previous, concurrent, or subsequent exposure to other chemicals, This fact has considerable importance in applied toxicology for man, economic animals, and domestic animals but is generally of less practical importance for feral animals. During a season pesticides are often used repetitively or more than one pesticide may be used simulataneously or in sequence, and it is also possible that therapeutic agents may be used at the time of exposure of pesticides.

The modifying effects of multiple exposure may be to increase or to diminish the acute toxicity (Murphy, 1969b) and there are a very large number of examples of both effects in the published literature (Ball *et al.*, 1954; Frawley *et al.*, 1957; Cook *et al.*, 1957 and 1958; DuBois, 1958 and 1961; Hewlett, 1960; Murphy and DuBois, 1958; Rosenberg and Coon, 1958; Murphy *et al.*, 1959; Knaak and O'Brien, 1960; Seume and O'Brien, 1960a and 1960b; Arterberry *et al.*, 1962; Triolo and Coon, 1963; Hart and Fouts, 1963; Casida *et al.*, 1963; Hart *et al.*, 1963; Gerboth and Schwabe, 1964; Brodeur and DuBois, 1964; Frawley, 1965; McPhillips, 1969; Menzer, 1970; Chapman and Leibman, 1971; Chadwick and Freal, 1972; Bass *et al.*, 1972; Lynch and Coon, 1972; Mayer *et al.*, 1972). In order to test for interactive effects, multiple exposure of experimental animals can be undertaken and the data obtained can be analysed by the methods described in Chapter 2. Useful information can be achieved by studies on some of the enzyme systems involved in the metabolism of the of the toxicants.

Pesticidal activity is sometimes increased by the inclusion of synergists in formulations or by the concurrent use of more than one pesticide. As well as affecting the response of the target pest, the synergist may also affect toxicity to non-target species. Piperonyl butoxide is commonly used to synergize insecticides, it has a low acute toxicity in relation to non-target species (Brown, 1970) and has little insecticidal activity on its own. Conney *et al.* (1972) examined the influence of piperonyl butoxide on microsomal enzymes in mice and found that it was a potent inhibitor, but in rats it required more than 100 times the mouse dose to produce the same effect whereas in man the same investigators found that 0.71 mg/kg, by mouth, did not produce any evidence of microsomal enzyme inhibition.

$$H_2C\underset{O}{\overset{O}{<}}\underbrace{\qquad}_{}\overset{CH_2CH_2CH_3}{\underset{CH_2OCH_2CH_2OCH_2CH_2OC_4H_9}{}}$$

Piperonyl butoxide

Ectoparasite control on dogs and cats is sometimes achieved by the continuous use of insecticide impregnated collars. There has been concern that this continuous exposure of cats and dogs to low doses of pesticide could influence their response to anaesthetics or to other therapeutic agents. In the case of one of the most commonly used pesticides for this purpose, dichlorvos, there have been extensive interaction studies in dogs (Elsea *et al.*, 1970; Ritter *et al.*, 1970; Young *et al.*, 1970) and in cats (Albert *et al.*, 1974), and with both species the influence of the dichlorvos on subsequent exposure to other chemicals appears to have been negligible. The toxicity of dichlorvos to dogs has been described in detail by Snow (1973) and Snow and Watson (1973) and to cats by Allen *et al.* (1978); thus any interactive effects due to dichlorvos and other chemicals are easy to confirm. Other pesticides used for this type of ectoparasite control (e.g. pyrethrum, tetrachlorvinphos, etc) have been less investigated for their possible effects on the toxicity of other concurrently administered chemicals but there has been no evidence of adverse effects from actual use.

CHAPTER 5

Exposure as a hazard and the various routes of exposure

EXPOSURE AS A HAZARD

By definition pesticides are intended to be toxic to target organisms. Unfortunately, to a greater or lesser extent pesticides are also toxic to non-target species although the relationship between the desirable and the undesirable toxicities is very variable. Exposure of non-target organisms may occur either deliberately or adventitiously.

A. Deliberate lethal exposure

(i) Suicide

Suicide is peculiar to man and misuse of pesticides for the purpose is not uncommon. Many pesticides are extremely toxic to man and may be readily obtained for this illicit use (Mant, 1960; Simpson, 1964; Gitelson *et al.*, 1965; Namba *et al.*, 1971; Dudley and Thaoar, 1972; Lisella, 1972; Lewin and Love, 1974; Lautenschläger *et al.*, 1974; Amarasingahm and Ti Thiow Hee, 1976).

(ii) Murder and manslaughter

Pesticides have been effectively used for murder and manslaughter and there are many well-documented cases in the forensic literature (Mant, 1960; Simpson, 1964; Namba *et al.*, 1971; Lisella, 1972; Amarasingahm and Ti Thiow Hee, 1976; Emsley, 1978); again the ease with which some of these toxic chemicals can be obtained is an important contributory factor.

(iii) Pest control

Some vertebrate pests may be legitimately controlled by the use of toxic chemicals (Turtle and Taylor, 1955; Peregrine, 1973). However, pesticides for this purpose should be very specific in their action (Roszkowski, 1965 and 1967; Cornwell and Bull, 1967; Cornwell, 1969; Gratz, 1973) and too many non-specific pesticides are used for this purpose thus presenting a serious hazard to non-target species (Bennett, 1972; Smith and Boyd, 1972; Lees, 1972). For example, the World Health Organization has strongly recommended against the use of thallium sulphate (Emsley, 1978) as a rodenticide on the basis of its known hazard to non-target species including man (World Health Organization Technical Report Series number 512, 1973); in the same report there is a recommendation that the selective rodenticide phosazetim should not be used at all because it has been shown to be neurotoxic to some species.

$$\left[Cl-\!\!\left\langle \bigcirc \right\rangle\!\!-O- \right]_2 \begin{array}{c} P-NH-C=NH \\ \| \quad\quad | \\ S \quad\quad CH_3 \end{array}$$

Phosazetim

There are occasions when highly toxic non-specific pesticides may be used under strictly controlled conditions for specific purposes. This has been done in nature reserves to protect the eggs of rare birds from predators; this approach has also been used to control rabid animals in areas where rabies is endemic. The use of attractive bait filled with highly toxic pesticides (e.g. eggs filled with strychnine) to kill vermin is common practice in many rural communities and can represent a very serious hazard to man and other animals (Kelsey, 1971). In Australia the so-called 'Tarbaby' technique makes use of the behaviour pattern of the target pest for killing rabbits; rabbits habitually lick their paws thereby absorbing sodium fluoroacetate that has been picked up from a treatment of the ground near the warrens. The amount of sodium fluoroacetate used to treat the ground is generally safe for man and other animals that do not lick their feet (Myers, 1976).

Strychnine

The malicious killing of animals, such as pets, by the misuse of pesticides is known to occur (Rogers *et al.*, 1973).

There are examples of chemicals intended for use against one class of pests being used successfully for the control of pests from entirely different classes. The insecticide parathion is used to kill the avian pest the weaver bird (*Quelea quelea*) in parts of Africa (Crook and Ward, 1968; Pope and Ward, 1972; Ward, 1973) and the insecticide endrin is commonly used to kill rodents (Petrella *et al.*, 1975). Although not pest control, a comparable use of pesticides to kill animals for food purposes is well known. Derris and rotenone or the extracts of flowers containing chemicals related to them have been used for many years to kill fish for human consumption (Loeb and Engstrom-Heg, 1970). These particular insecticides are highly piscicidal but have a low toxicity to mammals (Fukami *et al.*, 1970).

Endrin

B. Deliberate non-lethal exposure

Vertebrate animals are sometimes exposed deliberately to pesticides although they may not be the target organism. Such occasions are:

(i) Therapeutic exposure

Ectoparasites on animals, including man, are commonly eradicated by means of pesticides. There have been human tragedies due to over-exposure to insecticides used as shampoos for extoparasite control and the majority of these have involved parathion (Metcalf, 1957; Koeffler, 1958; Cann, 1963). Other animals have also been affected by this type of exposure.

No amount of predictive testing will prevent the type of disaster occasioned by the careless use of the wrong pesticide as for example the farmer who killed many head of cattle by using an unlabelled container of demeton while assuming it to be DDT (Watson *et al.*, 1971).

Sometimes pesticides are administered systemically to treat host animals for ectoparasite infestation (e.g. fenchlorphos for parasitic mites) but even more commonly pesticides are administered for endoparasitic diseases in both man and other vertebrate animals (e.g. anthelmintics, ascaricides, coccidiostats, etc.).

An example of a therapeutic use for a pesticide was the administration of dinitro-*o*-cresol (DNOC), a herbicide, for the purpose of slimming in humans (Brody, 1955). This use is no longer recommended and is considered to be very dangerous (Harvey *et al.*, 1951; Parker *et al.*, 1951; Bidstrup *et al.*, 1952; King and Harvey, 1953).

DNOC (dinitro-*o*-cresol)

(ii) *Diagnostic exposure*

Occasionally the exhibition of signs of a sensitization reaction, such as acute contact dermatitis or asthma, has tempted clinicians to carry out diagnostic tests with pesticides as the suspect allergens. Because of the small amounts of pesticides used in these tests they are freqeuntly accomplished without adverse sequelae, however, great care is needed with some of the more toxic materials used as pesticides. Bell *et al.* (1968) described a near fatality caused by diagnostic patch tests carried out with the organophosphorus insecticide mevinphos.

C. Adventitious exposure

At all stages during the manufacture, formulation, and packaging of pesticides, and sometimes during the actual use, the possibility of adventitious exposure is great (Metcalf, 1957; Nelson, 1977). Control rests with the adequacy of the occupational hygiene and this, in turn, is related to the knowledge and understanding of the chemistry, physical properties, and toxicology of the materials being handled (Rodnitzky *et al.*, 1975). Valuable information on the toxicity of pesticides can be obtained retrospectively by studying occupationally exposed people from manufacturing and formulation plants (Kazantzis *et al.*, 1964; Laws *et al.*, 1967; Jager, 1970) or from agricultural workers (Hayes Jr., 1959 and 1971; Durham and Wolfe, 1962; Wolfe *et al.*, 1966 and 1967; Lloyd and Bell, 1967; Durham *et al.*, 1972; Starr and Clifford, 1972); on occasions the information obtained in this manner may be surprising, as for example the fatality reported after a powder formulation of the insecticide malathion, with its apparently favourable acute toxicity (Gaines, 1960; Weeks *et al.*, 1977), blew into the respiratory tract of a man who was opening a container (Sellassie and Lester, 1971) and the incidence of acute toxicity reported for spraymen in some areas associated with the same insecticide (Shihab, 1976; Baker *et al.*, 1978).

Despite knowledge of the acute toxicity of pesticides, fatalities do occur occasionally with agricultural and horticultural workers (Hayes Jr., 1975 and 1977).

There are various international regulations to minimize the hazard of pesticide transportation by land, sea or air but accidents do occur and acute toxicity may be a hazard. For example the contamination of flour being transported in close proximity to the insecticide endrin (Davies and Lewis, 1956; Weeks, 1967) and cloth used for bedding and clothing contaminated with parathion during transport (Anderson *et al.*, 1965). The enforcement of transport regulations is difficult and not always successful (Stringer, 1968). Even when the law is complied with, accidents such as ships sinking, road and rail tankers overturning, or aeroplanes crashing can release toxicants into the environment with serious consequences.

The disposal of unwanted pesticides and pesticide-contaminated containers can present serious toxicity problems (Ganelin *et al.*, 1964b;

Watson *et al.*, 1971; Gehlback and Williams, 1975). Sometimes the use of pesticide waste or the disposal of pesticide intermediates can cause problems of acute toxicity (Editorial, *Fd. Cosmet. Toxicol.*, 1964; Coleman-Cooke, 1965). Kimbrough *et al.* (1977) reported an incident in which a great many horses and other animals were killed in the Eastern Missouri area of the U.S.A. by the spraying of waste oil from a manufacturing plant, the oil contained a highly toxic tetrachloro-benzodioxin.

Tetrachlorobenzodioxins

Personnel associated with the application of pesticides are particularly vulnerable to accidental exposure (Durham and Wolfe, 1962; Wolfe *et al.*, 1966 and 1967; Lloyd and Bell, 1967; Wolfe, 1972a and 1972b; Sellassie and Lester, 1971; Nagata, 1972; Durham *et al.*, 1965 and 1972). Although it is relatively easy to advise on the safety precautions to be used by personnel it is far more difficult to ensure that the advice is heeded. The climate in many areas in which pesticides are particularly necessary may preclude the wearing of impermeable protective clothing and, because of the dangers of overheating, the wearing of protective clothing may be more dangerous than the hazard associated with exposure to the pesticide (Wolfe, 1972a and 1972b; Matthews and Clayphon, 1973). Even where protective clothing is provided and wearable there is a common misconception that waterproof materials will necessarily be impermeable to other chemicals; this is not only wrong but dangerous, for it is possible that some toxic chemicals may penetrate the material of the clothing and build up dangerous concentrations of toxicant in contact with the skin (Locati *et al.*, 1968; Weber and Berencsi, 1972). Footwear can be critical, for example there are recorded deaths in pesticide workers because of concentrates spilling onto canvas shoes (Wolfe, 1972b) and Reichert *et al.* (1978) have reported the case of a sprayman wearing full protective clothing but who managed to get mevinphos and parathion into his boots.

In addition to protective clothing there are many other devices for the protection of personnel (e.g. respirators, dust masks, enclosed cabins for tractors, etc.). The whole subject of protective clothing and other safety equipment for use with pesticides has received intensive attention in some places.[a]

The time interval to be imposed between the application of a pesticide

[a]*Proceedings of the National Conference on Protective Clothing and Safety Equipment for Pesticide Workers* (Federal Working Group on Pest Management), Rockville, Md., U.S.A. – 1972.

and the entry of people and domestic animals into the treated area is very important and varies for different locations, different pesticides, and for different crops. The study of these re-entry times has become very important (Serat, 1973); they are investigated by means of predictive animal tests (Guthrie *et al.*, 1974; Skinner and Kilgore, 1978), human experience (Ware *et al.*, 1973 and 1974), and mathematical analysis (Serat *et al.*, 1975) in order to provide practical guidelines for use.

Animals, both wild and domesticated, are also vulnerable to adventitious exposure to pesticides (Allcroft and Jones, 1969; Allcroft *et al.*, 1969; Bennett, 1972; Smith and Boyd, 1972; Lloyd, 1973; Hilbery *et al.*, 1973; Wilkinson, 1973; Udall, 1973; Stevenson and Carter, 1975; Carbone *et al.*, 1976). Animals may be exposed under the same circumstances as man but additionally, because of their eating habits, both domestic and wild animals are particularly vulnerable to bait formulations (Davis, 1970; Bell, 1972; Udall, 1973; Stevenson and Carter, 1975). Wild animals cannot always be protected from the hazards of pesticides but careful programming of pesticide application schemes can often minimize the danger (Blackmore, 1963; Bell, 1972; Wiese *et al.*, 1973; Pillmore, 1973). Even so, the vagaries of natural events can upset the pattern; for example, exceptional weather conditions have been suggested as the cause of wild geese in Scotland and parts of Northern England digging up cereal and eating the seeds that had been treated with carbophenothion, with fatal results (Hamilton *et al.*, 1976). Photolysis of pesticides may change their toxicity after application (Khan *et al.*, 1973).

An example of the 'food-chain effect' manifesting itself as an acute intoxication in birds has been reported (Jones, 1977). Owls in an aviary were fed on killed mice that had been bred and maintained on sawdust. The sawdust originated from a timber company that also supplied dieldrin-treated wood for the manufacture of window frames and quite clearly the use of dieldrin-impregnated wood for the production of sawdust for use in animal husbandry is not recommended by the pesticide manufacturers. Although the mice appeared to be normal and healthy when alive, the residues of the insecticide in their bodies were sufficient to kill the owls. Dieldrin in wood shavings has been responsible for poultry deaths when used in the deep-litter system (Amure and Stuart, 1978; Taylor, 1978) and pentachlorophenol, a wood preservative, has also been implicated in acute intoxications involving sawdust (Munro *et al.*, 1977). An example of acute intoxication occurring as a result of a food-chain effect in humans occurred in New Mexico when pigs were fed grain that had been treated with an organomercurial and were then used for meat (Curley *et al.*, 1971).

Normal agricultural practice may put individuals or communities at risk (Sachsse and Hess, 1972; Simpson and Penney, 1974). Spray drift, often due to changes in wind direction during the spraying operation, has sometimes caused people in nearby locations to be exposed to pesticides

(Luckmann and Decker, 1960; Gardner and Iverson, 1968; Arnan, 1971; Klemmer, 1972). The crew of spraying aircraft can be affected causing errors of judgement (Borredon, 1970; Clark, 1971; Wood et al., 1971), and pain can follow accidents involving pesticides (McLeod, 1975).

People entering pesticide-treated areas before the appropriate 're-entry time' has elapsed may be intoxicated by contact (Quinby and Lemmon, 1958; Hegazy, 1965; Ware et al., 1973 and 1974).

Many dangerous pesticides can be handled by experts but are a serious hazard when made available to lay-people. The herbicide paraquat has been the cause of numerous fatalities (Bullivant, 1966; Duffy and O'Sullivan, 1968; Weidenbach, 1969; McDonaugh and Martin, 1970; Masterson and Roche, 1970); several of these were due to the stupidity of people sub-packaging the product in bottles associated with consumable drinks. This same stupidity has been the cause of death with some other pesticides (Munoz-Villegas and Carcur-Giacaman, 1971).

The consumption of foodstuffs containing excessive amounts of pesticides can be acutely hazardous (Coble et al., 1967). Grain treated with organomercurial seed-dressings and intended only for planting has, on several occasions, been eaten with disasterous results (Davies and Lewis, 1956; Jalili and Abbasi, 1961; Taylor et al., 1969; Damluji and Tikriti, 1972; Barnes, 1973; Derban, 1974). Other foodstuffs contaminated by pesticides during transit (e.g. owing to leaking drums of pesticide in the hold of a ship etc.) have also been the cause of intoxication. The storage of pesticides in food containers, whether labelled or not, is highly dangerous (De Palma et al., 1970).

Adventitious exposure of people can occur during the misuse of pesticides during hostilities (Yegiazarov, 1971). It has been estimated (Handler, 1974) that about 200 to 300 lb of the highly toxic impurity 2,3,7,8-tetrachlorodibenzo-p-dioxin mixed with about 50 000 000 lb of the herbicide 2,4,5-T was sprayed during the defoliation programme during the hostilities in South Vietnam.

Fire in buildings or transport associated with pesticides can be very hazardous. Frequently pesticides are formulated in inflammable solvents thus increasing the fire risk and with the added danger of an explosion further spreading the toxicant. In many such cases, heat may cause the volatilization of pesticides into toxic vapours. Some organophosphorus compounds can be converted by pyrolysis into highly toxic cyclic phosphate esters (Bellet and Casida, 1973). The hazards associated with fire and pesticides have been reviewed by McSmith and Ledbetter (1971) and by Benson (1973).

Children and adults have been affected by contact with contaminated clothing and bedding (Quinby and Lemmon, 1958; Anderson et al., 1965) and footwear (Reichert et al., 1978), thus emphasizing the need for thorough decontamination procedures.

Unsuitable storage conditions can alter the acute toxicity potential of

D

some pesticides (Umetsu *et al*., 1977). In 1976 some 7 500 field workers in the Pakistan malaria control programme were affected by malathion that had been stored under conditions that gave rise to the more toxic isomalathion (Baker Jr. *et al*., 1978).

CH$_3$O, S
   P
CH$_3$O   S—CH—COOC$_2$H$_5$
              |
              CH$_2$—COOC$_2$H$_5$

Malathion

CH$_3$S, O
   P
CH$_3$O   S—CH—COOC$_2$H$_5$
              |
              CH$_2$—COOC$_2$H$_5$

iso-Malathion

EXPOSURE IN PREDICTIVE TOXICOLOGICAL TESTING

Predictive toxicological testing for the assessment of acute effects with pesticides utilizes the common routes of exposure (i.e. ingestion from the alimentary tract, absorption through the skin and to a much less extent the eyes, and also absorption following inhalation). Parenteral administration is also used because this can provide valuable information on the metabolism and distribution of the toxicants (Ramachandran, 1966; Natoff, 1967; Walsh and Fink, 1972). There are reviews of pharmacokinetics and pharmaco-dynamics that are relevant to acute toxicity (Keberle, 1971; O'Reilly, 1972), and a discussion of some of these aspects follows:

Ingestion

Ingestion is generally referred to as 'oral' or 'peroral' exposure and includes direct intragastric exposure in experimental acute toxicology.

The buccal cavity

Because of the rich blood supply to the mucous membranes of the mouth, many compounds can be absorbed through them (Moffat, 1971; Beckett and Hossie, 1971). Absorption from the buccal cavity is limited to unionized lipid-soluble compounds. Buccal absorption of a wide range of aromatic and aliphatic acids and basic drugs in human subjects has been found to be parabolically dependent on log P, when P is the octanol–water partition coefficient. The ideal lipophilic character (log P_o) for maximum buccal absorption has also been shown to be in the range 4.2–5.5 (Lien *et al*., 1971). Compounds with large molecular weights are poorly absorbed in the buccal cavity and, since absorption increases linearly with concentration and there is no discrimination between optical enantiomorphs of several compounds known to be absorbed from the mouth, it is believed that uptake of toxicants is by passive diffusion rather than active transport (Beckett and Hossie, 1971).

A knowledge of the buccal absorption characteristics of a pesticide can be important for in the case of accidental poisoning it is possible that, although the toxicant taken into the mouth is voided on being found objectionable, significant absorption may already have occurred before any material has been swallowed.

The gastro-intestinal tract

Unless voided, most materials from the buccal cavity are swallowed and enter the gastro-intestinal tract. No significant absorption occurs in the oesophagus and the toxicant passes on to enter the stomach. It is common practice in acute toxicity testing to avoid the possibility of buccal absorption by administering the toxicant directly into the stomach by intra-oesophageal intubation (N.B. This technique is often referred to as 'gavage') or by the administration of the toxicant in gelatine capsules designed to disintegrate in the gastric fluid.

Absorption of chemicals with widely different characteristics can occur at different levels in the gastro-intestinal tract (Schanker, 1960). The two factors most influencing this absorption are:

(a) The lipid–water partition characteristics of the undissociated toxicant.
(b) The dissociation constant which determines the amount of toxicant in the dissociated form.

Hence, weak organic acids and bases are readily absorbed as uncharged lipid-soluble molecules whereas ionized compounds are absorbed only with difficulty and unionized toxicants with poor lipid-solubility characteristics are absorbed slowly.

Lipid-soluble acid molecules can be absorbed efficiently through the gastric mucosa but bases are not absorbed in the stomach.

In the intestines the unionized form of the toxicant is preferentially absorbed and rate of absorption is related to the lipid–water partition coefficient of the toxicant. The highest pK_a value for a base compatible with efficient gastric absorption is about 7.8 and the lowest pK_a for an acid is about 3.0, although a limited amount of absorption can occur outside these pK_a values. Houston *et al.* (1974) investigated the gastric absorption and the intestinal absorption of a series of carbamates with different carbon chain lengths; absorption from the stomach increased as the chain lengthened from methyl to *n*-hexyl whereas intestinal absorption increased over the range methyl to *n*-butyl and then diminished as the chain length further increased. These investigators concluded that to explain the logic of optimal partition coefficients for intestinal absorption it was necessary to postulate a two-compartment model with a hydrophilic barrier and a lipoidal membrane and that if there is an acceptable optimal partition coefficient for gastric absorption it must be at least ten times greater than the corresponding intestinal value. In a further series of experiments, the same investigators, Houston *et al.* (1975), working with seven

N-methylated carbamates confirmed the difference in partition characteristics required for gastric and for intestinal absorption.

Carbaryl, a very lipophilic insecticidal carbamate, has been shown to be efficiently absorbed in many species of animal including man (Wills *et al.*, 1968); however Pekas and Giles (1974) have demonstrated that gastric contents can diminish the absorption of carbaryl and can allow metabolism of the compound to occur in the gastro-intestinal tract.

$$O.CO.NH.CH_3$$

Carbaryl

The rate of absorption of toxicants from the gastro-intestinal tract can be critical to the outcome of intoxication and this has major implications in respect of the formulation of pesticides and also to antidote therapy.

The state of fullness of the gastro-intestinal tract (Hunt, 1963; Doluisio *et al.*, 1969a and 1969b) and the nature of the contents (Schanker, 1960; Miller *et al.*, 1966; Boyd, 1972), the gastric emptying rate (Hunt, 1963; Maeda *et al.*, 1977), as well as the presence of products having an effect on the mucosa or on the blood supply to the tract (Winne, 1970; Riegelman and Rowland, 1974) can all significantly affect absorption. Doluisio *et al.* (1969a and 1969b) demonstrated that in an *in situ* rat intestinal preparation, no apparent deviation in absorption patterns occurred when fasting periods were less than 20 hours but if the fasting time exceeded 20 hours absorption rates decreased significantly in a time-dependent way. Worden and Harper (1964) and van Harken and Hottendorf (1978) demonstrated the effect of some of these factors on toxicant absorption and Boyd (1972) investigated the effect of these and other factors on the absorption of some toxicants and nutrients. Prescott *et al.* (1977) have reviewed the various interactions that may occur to affect absorption of chemicals when multiple exposures occur.

Several mechanisms are involved in the process of absorption from the gastro-intestinal tract:

(i) Passive absorption The lining membrane of the tract has a passive role. As toxicant molecules move from the bulk water phase of the intestinal contents into the epithelial cells, they must pass through two membranes in series, one is a layer of water and the other the lipid membrane of the microvillus surface (Wilson and Dietschy, 1974). The water layer may be the absolutely rate-limiting factor for passive absorption into the intestinal mucosa but it is not rate limiting for active absorption (see (ii) and (iii) below). The concentration gradient as well as the physico-chemical properties of the toxicant and of the lining membrane

are the controlling factors. Pesticides that are highly lipid-soluble are capable of passive diffusion and they pass readily from the aqueous fluids of the gut lumen through the lipid barrier of the intestinal wall and into the bloodstream. The interference in the absorption process by the water layer increases with increasing absorbability of the substances in the intestine (Winne, 1978).

Aliphatic carbamates are rapidly absorbed from the colon by passive uptake (Wood *et al.*, 1978) and it is found that there is a linear relationship between log k_a and log P for absorption of these carbamates in the colon and the stomach whereas there is a parabolic relationship between these two values for absorption in the small intestine (Houston *et al.*, 1975). The variables quoted are:

$$P = \text{octanol–buffer partition coefficient}$$

$$k_a = \text{absorption rate constant} \quad \frac{\ln 2}{t^{1/2}}$$

$$t = \text{time}$$

Organic acids that are ionized at intestinal pH are absorbed by simple diffusion (Lanman *et al.*, 1971) and Hwang and Schanker (1973) found that pentavalent arsenical compounds are slowly absorbed in the same way.

(ii) Facilitated diffusion Temporary combination of the toxicant with some form of 'carrier' occurs in the gut wall and the transfer of the toxicant across the membranes is facilitated. This process is also dependent on the concentration gradient across the membrane and there is no energy utilization in making the translocation. In some intoxications the 'carrier' may become saturated and this can be a rate-limiting step in the absorption process.

(iii) Active transport As in (ii), the process depends on a 'carrier', but differs in that the 'carrier' provides energy for translocation from regions of lower electrochemical potential to regions of higher potential.

(iv) Pinocytosis This is the process by which particles are absorbed and can be an important factor with the ingestion of particular formulations of pesticides (e.g. dust formulations, suspensions of wettable powders etc.), although it must not be confused with the absorption by one of the above processes of toxicant that has been released from the particles.

(v) Absorption via lymphatic channels Some lipophilic chemicals may be absorbed through the lymphatics dissolved in lipids.

(vi) Convective absorption Compounds with molecular radii of less than 4 nm can pass through pores in the gut membrane. The membrane exhibits a sieving effect.

Characteristically, within certain concentration limits, if a toxicant is absorbed by passive diffusion (i), then the concentration of toxicant in the gut and the rate of absorption are linearly related. However, if absorption is mediated by active transport (iii), the relationship between concentration and rate of absorption conforms to Michaelis–Menten kinetics and a Lineweaver–Burk plot (i.e. reciprocal of rate of absorption plotted against reciprocal concentration) gives a straight line.

Differences in the physiological chemistry of the gastro-intestinal fluids can have a significant effect on toxicity. Both physical and chemical differences in the gastro-intestinal tract can lead to species differences in susceptibility to acute intoxication. The anthelmintic pyrvinium chloride has an identical LD_{50} value when administered intraperitoneally to rats and mice (approximately 4 mg/kg) but when administered orally the LD_{50} value to mice was found to be 15 mg/kg although for the rat the LD_{50} values were 430 mg/kg for females and 1 550 mg/kg for males; it is thought that this is an absorption difference rather than a metabolic difference (Roszkowski, 1967). The rodenticide zinc phosphide depends for its action on the release of phosphine by interaction of the phosphide with hydrochloric acid in the stomach (Johnson and Voss, 1952); thus dogs and cats are more resistant to zinc phosphide intoxication than are rats and rabbits since the former secrete gastric hydrochloric acid only intermittently whereas the latter secrete acid almost continuously.

Pyrvinium chloride

By increasing or decreasing the viscosity of a formulation the absorption of a toxicant can be altered (Ritschel et al., 1974). Fincher (1968) has defined some of the physico-chemical aspects of absorption of toxicants from particulate formulations in the gastro-intestinal tract. Conversely, the use of inert adsorbents to diminish absorption has been used as antidote therapy for some forms of intoxication. This approach to treatment has been studied in detail following acute exposure to the herbicide paraquat (Clark, 1971; Staiff et al., 1973; Smith et al., 1974). With the knowledge that rats cannot vomit, there have been serious attempts at making rodenticides safer to non-target animals by incorporating emetics into the formulations but this has had only a limited success.

Most of any toxicant absorbed from the gastro-intestinal tract must pass through the liver via the hepatic-portal venous system (Gibaldi et al., 1971; Riegelman and Rowland, 1974) and, as mixing of the venous blood with hepatic arterial blood occurs, care is needed in interpreting the amounts of toxicant both in the blood and in the liver. Gaines *et al.* (1966) used *in vivo* liver perfusion techniques to investigate the apparent anomaly that the carbamate ISOLAN was more toxic when administered to rats percutaneously that when administered orally (Gaines, 1960). It has been shown (Brown, 1968) that these results are a manifestation of different formulations having been used for the two routes of exposure and by estimating the LD_{50} values using a common solvent, *n*-octanol, for both routes of exposure it was found that ISOLAN was significantly more toxic by the oral route than by the percutaneous route (Table 5.1) and by regression analysis it was found that at no level of lethal dose values was the reverse correct.

Despite the gastro-intestinal absorption characteristics discussed above, it is common for absorption from the alimentary tract to be facilitated by dilution of the toxicant (Ferguson, 1962; Borowitz *et al.*, 1971). Borowitz *et al.* (1971) have suggested that the concentration effects that they observed with atropine sulphate, aminopyrine, sodium salicylate, and sodium pentobarbital were due to a combination of rapid stomach emptying and the large surface area for absorption of the drugs. Kodama (personal communication), during investigations of the pharmacological properties of some symmetrical triazines, demonstrated an inverse relationship between efficacy and concentration of an oral dose of the experimental compound DW 2172/WL 11828-D in mice; he further showed that the volume of gastric secretion and gastric acid production was reduced after oral administration of DW 2172/WL 11828-D to rats.

Since some *s*-triazines have a direct pharmacological effect on the alimentary tract (Kodama—unpublished), it is probable that absorption may as a result be affected and hence there will be variations in the acute toxicity. The author and co-workers (Brown *et al.*—unpublished data) have shown that the symmetrical triazine herbicide atrazine is more acutely toxic to rats when administered in dilute solutions or suspension than when administered in a more concentrated form. Similar studies with two related herbicides, cyanazine and simazine, indicate that the magnitude of the response to atrazine may be exceptional.

This finding that decreasing concentration of toxicant in a vehicle may increase its intrinsic toxicity illustrates the problem associated with legislative categorization of pesticides on the basis of LD_{50} values.

Table 5.1 The acute oral and percutaneous LD_{50} values for ISOLAN administered to rats as a solution in n-octanol

LD_{50} mg/kg	(95% confidence limits)
Oral	Percutaneous
4.5 (3.2–6.1)	7.2 (5.6–9.2)

$$\text{Cl}$$

(Triazine ring structure)

$$R^1HN \quad NHR^2$$

	R^1	R^2
Atrazine	$-Et$	$-isoPr$
Cyanazine	$-Et$	$-CMe_2CN$
Simazine	$-Et$	$-Et$

$$CCl_3$$

(Triazine ring structure with morpholine)

$$ON \quad N \quad NH.CH_2CH_2OH$$

DW 2172/WL 11828-D

Major structural or physiological differences in the alimentary tract (e.g. species differences or surgical effects) can give rise to modifications of toxicity. For example, ruminant animals may exhibit metabolism of toxicants in the gastro-intestinal tract in a way that is unlikely to occur in non-ruminants (Radeleff, 1970; Clarke and Clarke, 1975).

The presence of bile salts in the alimentary tract can affect absorption of toxicants in a variety of ways (Kakemi et al., 1970).

Absorption through the skin (dermal exposure; percutaneous absorption)

Contamination of the skin with subsequent absorption of the toxicant is undoubtedly the major form of accidental or adventitious acute exposure to pesticides.[b]

Adventitious exposure to pesticide formulations during handling and application are common (Fristedt and Sterner, 1965; Lloyd and Bell, 1967; Wolfe et al., 1966 and 1967; Simpson and Simpson, 1969; Durham et al., 1972).

Sometimes the skin exposure may be deliberate as for example the use of pesticides for ectoparasite control in man and other animals (Pickering, 1965; Walker and Stevenson, 1968; Grover, 1971). Deliberate percutaneous exposure of man to pesticides for clinical diagnostic purposes is rare but not unknown (Bell et al., 1968) whereas deliberate, controlled exposure of human skin in vivo to pesticides for experimental purposes is

---

[b]Proceedings of the National Conference on Protective Clothing and Safety Equipment for Pesticide Workers (Federal Working Group in Pest Management) Rockville, MD, U.S.A. – 1972.

not uncommon (Elliott *et al.*, 1960; Funckes *et al.*, 1963; Hayes *et al.*, 1964; Hunter, 1969; Maibach *et al.*, 1970 and 1971; Feldmann and Maibach, 1974).

The deliberate exposure of animals to pesticides for the investigation of percutaneous hazard is a frequent occurrence. These tests may fall into two distinct, but related, types. Firstly, there are those tests designed to investigate the ability of a pesticide to penetrate the skin on the basis of the physico-chemical properties of either the pesticide or its formulation (Draize *et al.*, 1944; Johnston and Eden, 1953; Cartter, 1961; Kundiev, 1963 and 1965; Vandekar and Komanov, 1963; Vandekar *et al.*, 1963; Medved and Kundiev, 1964; Brown, V. K. H., 1964, 1965, and 1968; Brown and Muir, 1971; O'Brien and Dannelley, 1965; Marzulli *et al.*, 1965; Bojanowska and Brzezicka-Bak, 1967). There are also percutaneous exposure tests intended to give some measure of hazard (Gaines, 1960 and 1969; Weil *et al.*, 1971), data of this latter type occur throughout the literature for individual pesticides as they form an essential part of the overall toxicological assessment for all pesticides.

There are five routes of percutaneous entry for toxicants (Marzulli, 1962; Scheuplein, 1965 and 1967):

  (i) Between the cells of the stratum corneum;
 (ii) Through the cells of the stratum corneum;
(iii) Via the hair follicles;
(iv) Via the sweat glands;
 (v) Via the sebaceous glands.

The existence of a specific barrier zone in the epidermis is a matter for controversy. The idea of a specific barrier layer in the epidermis was postulated some years ago but its physical isolation from human skin is attributed to Szakall (1951), hence it is sometimes called the 'Szakall layer'. Mali (1956) demonstrated that the 'Szakall layer' may not be functionally simple, later Buettner (1963) utilized the data of both Szakall and Mali together with his own physical methods to study transepidermal water movement and postulated that there are two barrier zones. The same year Onken and Moyer (1963) found that the barrier layer could be extracted chemically, giving rise to an increase in skin permeability, and Crounse (1965) demonstrated that the solvent-extracted material could be used to construct models for penetration studies *in vivo*.

By the use of histochemical techniques Wohlrab *et al.* (1967) demonstrated that a distinct barrier zone could be found in the intermediary part of the epidermis of human skin. Elias (1975), using water-soluble tracers and freeze-fracture techniques, found that the primary barrier to water-loss in the skin is formed in the stratum granulosum and is subserved by intercellular deposition of lamellar bodies rather than junctions and that percutaneous absorption of water-soluble materials through normal or disrupted stratum corneum occurs via the intercellular space. The same investigator (Elias, 1975) also found that solvent-treated skin exhibited some subcellular changes and that even severely damaged cornified cells never permitted penetration of water-soluble tracers.

Because of the widespread concern with the penetrability of toxicants some knowledge of the chemical nature of the barrier zone was needed. Blank and Scheuplein (1964) and Hicks (1966) established that the zone was composed of phospholipid material with associated sulphydryl and disulphide bridge groups. Elias *et al.* (1977) have further investigated the composition of the lipids involved in the barrier function. Cooke (1965) likened the barrier zone to an ionic sieve. If the epidermis is physically damaged its penetrability is substantially facilitated (Cronin and Stoughton, 1962), earlier Marzulli and Tregear (1961) had found that tri-*n*-propyl phosphate penetrated stripped human skin more easily than normal human skin. A comparable situation occurs when the skin is affected by some eczematous conditions (Starr and Clifford, 1971) and, because of sub-normal impedance, the eczematous skin behaves like stripped skin.

Opinions vary on the importance of the cutaneous appendages and ancillary structures as routes of absorption. Tregear (1962) suggested that the importance of the appendages was minimal whereas Grasso (1971) was of the opinion that the skin appendages formed an important pathway for both water-soluble and lipid-soluble chemicals.

The dynamic equilibrium between input through the skin and the fate of the toxicant is important. The rate of input may be profoundly influenced by the physical state of the toxicant and its mode of presentation to the skin (Brown, 1968). Lindsey (1962) and Blank and Scheuplein (1964) presented lists of factors that were considered critical to the subject of skin penetration; these lists can be summarized as follows:

(i) Small molecules penetrate skin better than large molecules.
(ii) Undissociated molecules penetrate skin better than do ions.
(iii) Preferential solubility of the toxicant in organic solvents indicates better penetration characteristics than preferential solubility in water.
(iv) The less viscous or the more volatile the toxicant the greater is its penetrating ability.
(v) The nature of the vehicle for the toxicant and the concentration of the toxicant in the vehicle both affect absorption.
(vi) The water content of the stratum corneum affects penetrability.
(vii) The ambient temperature can influence the uptake of toxicant through the skin.

It has been shown that some macromolecules such as albumin, dextrans, polyvinylpyrrolidone (Tregear, 1966b) and polypeptides (Kastin *et al.*, 1966) and even some colloids, can penetrate the barrier if the solvent system is favourable (Iunin, 1957).

Molecular shape has received little attention as a factor in skin penetration, but Medved and Kundiev (1964) suggested, with little supporting evidence, that molecular symmetry is important. Molecular weight and boiling point, but not molecular shape, were shown to correlate with the skin-penetrating properties of a series of trialkyl- and triaryl-phosphates by Marzulli *et al.* (1965), whereas for the same compounds there was an inverse relationship between octanol–water partition coefficients and the rate of skin penetration (Penniston *et al.*, 1969).

Transport of solvent or solute across biological membranes may be by one or more of three processes (Bray and White, 1966):

(a) Free diffusion;
(b) Carrier diffusion;
(c) Active transport.

In the skin, active transport is unimportant although it is possible to have a measurable active 'anti-transport'. 'Anti-transport' is apparent when skin enzymes react with the toxicant to partially or wholly inhibit penetration of unchanged chemical, Fredriksson *et al.* (1961) and Fredriksson (1964) showed that this could occur when paraoxon was applied to the skin. An analysis of this phenomenon has been carried out by Ando *et al.* (1977).

The skin is far too complex a barrier for simple free diffusion to be the principal mechanism of toxicant penetration although this process is undoubtedly involved to some extent (Kedem and Katchalsky, 1961).

The main process involved with skin penetration is carrier diffusion and, at low solute concentrations, it can be expected that the carrier will be mainly present in the free state and approximately proportional to the concentration of free solute. This being so, Fick's law of diffusion can be held to be approximately valid (Faucher and Goddard, 1978), although as Buerger (1967) has explained, this use of Fick's law can only be applied to the integument if intermolecular interactions are negligible. In the context of skin penetration, Fick's law may be written:

$$\frac{Q}{At} = F_s = K_p \, \Delta C_s$$

when,

Q = amount of solute that penetrates the skin (moles)

A = area of involved skin (cm^2)

t = time (s)

F_s = amount of solute penetrating per unit area of skin in unit time, or flux (mol cm^{-2} s^{-1})

K_p = permeability constant (cm s^{-1})

C_s = difference between concentrations of solute on both sides of the skin (mol cm^{-3})

Blank and Scheuplein (1964) and Scheuplein (1965) extended this by relating the flux to the epidermal thickness:

$$F_s = K_p \, \Delta \, C_s = \frac{KD}{d} \, \Delta \, C_s$$

or

$$K_p = \frac{DK}{d}$$

when,

K = partition coefficient

D = diffusion constant (cm^2 s^{-1})

d = epidermal thickness

But this simple relationship only holds good for single chemicals in contact with skin. For *in vivo* use, the permeability coefficient can be measured from excretion data provided that the excretion data are proportional to the concentration of the toxicant in the body fluids and that the asymptotic limit for the amount of material excreted is linear in time (Cooper, 1976). Blank and Scheuplein (1964) and Scheuplein (1965) carried out their investigations using a series of primary alcohols from methanol to *n*-octanol. Using *N*-octylamine, Cummings (1969) showed a concentration effect in relation to skin penetration but, with that compound, temperature was found to have a marked effect on the whole process because of the different physico-chemical interactions that occurred with the amine in contact with skin at different temperatures. These observations with *N*-octylamine indicate the strict limitations of the simple Fick's law approach to skin penetration studies.

Craig *et al.* (1977) investigated the uptake of the anticholinesterase agent VX (*s*-(*s*-di-isopropylaminoethyl)-*o*-ethyl methylphosphonothioate) by human skin *in vivo* and concluded that the storage of toxic materials in the skin is more of a problem if the contamination occurs in the cold because in moving with a warm environment rapid absorption from the depot occurs whereas if contamination occurs in a warm environment, depot formation is minimized and the skin can be cooled to form part of the decontamination procedure.

Apart from solvent–skin effect, it is possible for mixtures of chemicals to interact with skin differently from either chemical component alone and this combined effect may influence penetration. Dikshith *et al.* (1974) found that a mixture of the two insecticides Gamma-BHC and diazinon damaged the epidermis far more than either Gamma-BHC or diazinon alone. This is a further reason for being able to apply the Fick's law approach only to single toxicants.

$$CH_3$$

Diazinon

The diffusion constant (D) of a solute in the stratum corneum is a measure of the permeability of the stratum corneum. If the molecules of the solute are spherical and the molecules of the solvent are comparable or smaller in size, then the Stokes–Einstein equation will give an accurate measure of the value of D (Katz and Poulsen, 1971):

$$D = \frac{\beta T}{6 \eta r}$$

D = diffusion constant ($cm^2\ s^{-1}$)

β = Boltzmann constant ($1.380\ 3 \times 10^{-16}\ g\ cm^{-2}\ s^{-1}\ deg^{-1}$)

T = temperature (K)

r = hydrodynamic radius of the solute

η = viscosity of the stratum corneum

Thus, the diffusion constant decreases with increase in molecular weight, and the converse, and this leads to the conclusion that there will be a decrease in the rate of penetration with increase in molecular size. Using human skin in both *in vivo* and *in vitro* studies, Franz (1975) demonstrated a high degree of correlation between the penetrability of 12 unrelated chemicals (hippuric acid, nicotinic acid, nicotinamide, benzoic acid, salicylic acid, acetylsalicylic acid, thiourea, chloramphenicol, phenol, urea, caffeine, dinitrochlorobenzene) and their physical properties.

Because of the time required for a toxicant to pass through the epidermis and the magnitude of variation in epidermal thickness, the inclusion of a thickness factor in any mathematical relationship is a sound principle. Leider and Buncke (1954) measured the variation in thickness of epidermis in typical normal adult humans and found the range for most skin to be 0.07–0.17 mm, and the variation in total stratum corneum thickness varied over the range 0.03–0.05 mm. Using an improved measuring technique, Whitton and Everall (1973) confirmed that there is large variation in epidermal thickness in humans with an average of 0.04–0.05 mm for much of the body but achieving a thickness of 0.4 mm on the fronts of the fingers. Whitton and Everall (1973) found no correlation between epidermal thickness and age (N.B. they studied the range of ages 15–89 years), or between thickness and sex, but they found that environmental factors can influence the thickness.

Christophers and Kligman (1964) studied skin penetration in people aged 20–30 years and also in others aged over 68 years and they concluded that the skin of the older group was more permeable, but that there exists a compensatory impeded clearance due to decreased blood flow and connective tissue changes. Lee and Ng (1965) have demonstrated that above the age of 11 years, male humans possess a thicker skin than do comparable females. Maibach (1976—unpublished but quoted in *FDC Reports* **38** (No. 47) p. 16) has demonstrated by *in vitro* and *in vivo* techniques that the skin of new-born humans is not necessarily more permeable than the skin of adult humans. Solomon *et al.* (1977) measured the concentrations of the insecticide gamma-BHC in the blood and brain of guinea-pigs aged two months and also of new-born guinea-pigs, both groups having been exposed to the same percutaneous dose, the concentrations of insecticide found in the new-born animals were almost double those in the older ones.

Because the penetration rate differentials attributable to age and sex will generally be insignificant in relation to other factors (Lu *et al.*, 1965; Gaines, 1960 and 1969), these may be neglected in the assessment of the percutaneous toxicity of pesticides. Surface area of involved skin is also important; Blank and Scheuplein (1964) demonstrated that the water content of the stratum corneum from human skin increases under occlusive conditions to as much as 50%, from 5 to 15% in the normal non-occluded situation, but under identical conditions of occlusion Harris *et al.* (1974) have shown that the surface area may be increased by as much as 37%; this increase in area can be very important since most predictive tests in acute percutaneous toxicology are carried out with the toxicant applied to the skin under an occlusive dressing (Draize, 1959; Noakes and Sanderson, 1969).

In order to produce a systemic effect the skin penetrant must also enter the circulatory system. This can be a major source of discrepancy between penetrations *in vitro* and *in vivo*, but it can be shown that chemicals capable of passing the epidermal barrier zone can also be absorbed into capillaries. The subject of capillary permeability has been reviewed by Pappenheimer (1953). Application of the mathematical treatment of skin capillary absorption can be confounded when pesticides and their formulations are considered. For example, xylenes and trimethylbenzenes, both popular as solvents for pesticide formulations, can increase dermal capillary diameters and thus facilitate blood flow enormously (Aschheim, 1965; Brown and Box, 1971) and this will promote absorption into the circulation.

Although dilatation of the skin blood vessels facilitates absorption of compounds through the skin and into the systemic blood supply, there is no simple correlation between skin penetration and vasodilatation that is applicable to all materials.

In the context of vasodilatation temperature is also very important; human cutaneous circulation is dependent on the thermal balance of the subject and, in the cold, cutaneous blood flow may be less than 0.22 ml cm^{-2} min^{-1} while under conditions of heat stress it can rise to 0.3 ml cm^{-2} min^{-1} (Tregear, 1966).

It has sometimes been stated that the vehicle used is only of secondary importance to the lipid solubility of the solute when considering skin penetration (Rothman, 1943 and 1955; Ostrenga *et al.*, 1971) and further that if a chemical is not capable of passing the epidermal barrier, no vehicle will transport it across the barrier. Because *in vivo* there are numerous interacting factors these statements are an over-simplification, but for most practical purposes they are acceptable. The Overton–Meyer hypothesis (Mullins, 1954), relating water–lipid partition to narcotic properties may also be applicable when considering skin penetration and the water–lipid partition coefficient of the toxicant may be more important than its lipid solubility. This has been shown to be true for skin penetration by corticosteroids (Katz and Shaikh, 1965). Clendenning and Stoughton (1962) concluded that a water–lipid partition coefficient approaching unity was required for maximum skin penetration by weak electrolytes. However the situation is not quite so simple. Wurster and Dempski (1961) showed that absorption to the stratum corneum by the toxicant may confound the relationship between partition coefficient and penetration and that chemical interactions between the toxicant and the skin components, other than absorption, may also interfere (Roberts *et al.*, 1974). A reservoir effect can occur when some toxicants are in contact with skin and are capable of slow absorption (Scheuplein and Ross, 1974) and this was shown to occur with the highly lipophilic insecticide dieldrin (Negherbon, 1959).

HEOD
(dieldrin >85% HEOD)

Although the lipophilic compounds such as dieldrin can be absorbed efficiently from the dry state, toxic manifestations are accelerated by using solvents (Bojanowska and Brzezicka-Bak, 1967).

Ahdaya *et al.* (1978) compared the absorption rates for ten insecticides administered to mice orally in corn oil and percutaneously in acetone and concluded that penetration was approximately twice as rapid through the gastro-intestinal route as through the skin. In these experiments, Ahdaya *et al.* (1978) found that parathion and carbaryl penetrated most rapidly and dieldrin was the slowest of the compounds tested but also there was a general correlation for individual compounds through the two routes.

Marzulli *et al.* (1965) studied the skin penetration properties of a series of organic phosphates and they concluded that in the series of compounds investigated both aqueous and lipid solubility were essential for good penetration. Again there was a tendency to over-simplification. Multiple regression analysis of data from several sources, including that of Marzulli and his co-workers, led Lien and Tong (1973) to deduce that in addition to partition coefficients steric or electronic terms, such as molar refraction, Taft's polar substituent constant, and molecular weight, were all needed to improve correlation between chemicals and their skin-penetrating properties. Further, when the data of Marzulli *et al.* (1965) were subjected to rigorous mathematical interpretation by Penniston *et al.* (1969) it was found that the penetration rate had actually slowed down as the octanol–water partition coefficients of the chemicals had increased.

O'Brien and Dannelley (1965) carried out definitive absorption experiments using five radiolabelled insecticides (DDT, famphur, carbaryl, malathion, and dieldrin) in rats. These investigators demonstrated that there was considerable interference with any simple relationship between partition coefficient and skin penetration. O'Brien and Dannelley (1965) used three solvents for the five insecticides investigated and concluded that penetration rate for the toxicants increased in the order: corn oil, benzene, acetone.

$$CH_3O-\underset{\underset{O}{|}}{\overset{\overset{S}{\|}}{P}}-OCH_3$$

O=S=O

H$_3$C—N—CH$_3$

Famphur

A physico-chemical analysis of the percutaneous absorption process was devised by Higuchi (1960) and this included the value of activity coefficients. Later, Higuchi and Kinkel (1965) published a more detailed discussion of the derivation of solvent–solvent and solvent–solute interactions, with particular reference to the anticholinesterase agent sarin. Barrer (1941) derived equations for the calculation of the amount of material absorbed by diffusion from homogeneous distributions or solutions and Higuchi (1960) adapted some of this process to studies on inunction and mathematical models are still being developed for application in bio-pharmaceutics (Ayres and Laskar, 1974). Higuchi's formula can be expressed as:

$$Q = hCo \left[1 - \frac{8}{\pi^2} \sum_{m=0}^{\infty} \frac{1}{(2m+1)^2} \exp \left\{ \frac{-Dv(2m+1)^2 \pi^2 t}{4h^2} \right\} \right]$$

when,

Q = amount of toxicant absorbed at time t per unit area of exposure

Co = initial concentration of penetrating toxicant

Dv = diffusion constant of toxicant in solvent

t = elapsed time of application

h = thickness of applied phase

and the formula can be modified for toxicants that are present as suspensions in a vehicle (i.e. concentration is in excess of solubility):

$$Q = [(2Co - Cs)(CsDvt)]^{\frac{1}{2}}$$

If the solubility of the toxicant in the vehicle is very small (i.e. $Co \gg Cs$), the modified Higuchi equation can be simplified to:

$$Q = (2CoCsDvt)^{\frac{1}{2}}$$

Some toxicants may be present in significant amounts as vapours. The characteristics of percutaneous penetration of vapours are poorly defined (Kloche et al., 1963) although there has been considerable interest in the skin penetration of solvent vapours (Piotrowski, 1972; Riihimäki and Pfäffli, 1978). The organophosphorus anticholinesterase agent sarin has been studied as a liquid and as a vapour using excised human skin (Blank et al., 1957). It was concluded by Blank and his collaborators that penetration by the vapour was so slow that decomposition of the sarin occurred in the skin. A more stringent in vivo experiment by McPhail and Adie (1960), using rabbits as the test species, showed that with sarin vapour percutaneous absorption can be significant and that the general formula:

$$I = kA^{\alpha}C^{\beta}t^{s}$$

holds good when,

I = intake of sarin

A = area of skin exposed (cm^2)

C = vapour concentration (g m^{-3})

t = time of exposure (min)

α, β, s, are constants.

Under the conditions of the experiments the intake for each animal varied linearly with time but McPhail and Adie found that a very large variation in sarin intake occurred between rabbits.

Using an *in vitro* technique with nitrobenzene in the vapour phase, Lueck *et al*. (1957a and 1957b) made a model for vapour-phase skin penetration and found that the following equation could be applied to the data:

$$\text{Log}_{10}(Co - 2Cb) = (-2K/2.303)t + \log_{10} Co$$

when,

Co = concentration of vapour 'outside'

Cb = concentration of nitrobenzene 'inside'

K = permeability constant, determined by the application of Fick's law

For the purposes of the U.K. Pesticides Safety Precautions Scheme and also for the Council of Europe Registration of Pesticides Scheme, it is recommended that laboratory rats should be used for assessing acute percutaneous toxicity and that the exposure should be under an occlusive dressing (Noakes and Sanderson, 1969). The same recommendation occurs in the proposed EEC regulations for hazardous materials. In the U.S.A. and in some other countries, the rabbit is the most commonly used test species for acute percutaneous toxicity tests, the test material being applied under an occlusive dressing (Draize, 1959). By using 80 test materials with a wide range of acute toxicities, Weil *et al*. (1971) investigated the correlation between the acute toxicity values when the percutaneous toxicities were determined in rats after 4 hours exposure and in rabbits after 24 hours exposure, both under occlusive dressings. The investigators found that:

$$\text{Log}_{10} Y = 0.738\ 3(\log_{10} X - 0.148\ 0) - 0.303\ 8$$

when

Y = predicted 24 hour LD_{50} value for rabbits

X = actual 4 hour LD_{50} value for rats

The correlation value for that logarithmic data in the series of experiments was +0.8.

It is usual in the Noakes and Sanderson (1969) method with rats to utilize a 24 hour exposure period. Criticism of the use of covered exposure routinely has been expressed since it may give rise to unrealistically unfavourable data for some pesticides. McElligott (1972) found that this was particularly true for the quaternary herbicides paraquat and diquat when these products were applied to the skin as salts.

Unless the investigation of percutaneous toxicity is carried out in the species of ultimate interest the problems of extrapolation from one species to another are large. In addition to the basic species differences in toxicity (Carr, 1967; Rall, 1969; Dixon, 1976; Krasovskij, 1976) there are species differences in overall skin penetrability characteristics (Tregear, 1964) and also there are regional differences within each species (Maibach *et al.*, 1971). Tregear (1964) investigated the penetrability of the skins of rabbit, rat, pig, guinea-pig, and man *in vitro* with several different chemicals. With water, ethylene bromide or paraoxon dissolved in xylene, the skins of man and pig behaved in a similar manner, but with tri-*o*-tolyl phosphate human skin was very permeable whereas pig skin was almost impermeable. Tregear found that the converse of the tri-*o*-tolyl phosphate situation occurred with sodium ions (i.e. application of sodium chloride to the skin). In most of the investigations by Tregear (1964), the skin of the rat was more permeable than either human skin or pig skin and the skin of the guinea-pig tended to behave in a manner close to that of the skins of pigs and man. Rabbit skin *in vitro* was found to be very permeable to water.

Working with an unspecified organophosphorus compound, McCreesh (1965) demonstrated that the skins of the rat and of the rabbit were most readily penetrated and the skin of the pig least penetrated by the compound; other species lay between these extremes as follows: pig < dog < monkey = goat = cat < guinea-pig < rat = rabbit. Unfortunately human skin was not included in McCreesh's studies.

Whereas all the earlier comparative permeability studies were carried out by using *in vitro* techniques, Bartek *et al.* (1972) used radiolabelled compounds to investigate the absorption of six compounds through the skins of man, rabbit, rat, and pig. The six compounds had heptane–aqueous buffer partition coefficients ranging from 0.000 4 to 100.8. With one exception the rabbit skin was the most easily penetrated and the exceptional case, *N*-acetylcysteine (partition coefficient = 0.000 4), only penetrated any of the skins with difficulty. Bartek and his co-workers found that with the six compounds pig skin behaved in a similar manner to human skin and that both rat and rabbit skins were more readily penetrated. In the same laboratory Wester and Maibach (1975) investigated the skin penetration characteristics of three compounds, testosterone, hydrocortisone, and benzoic acid, in the rhesus monkey (*Macaca mulatta*) and man and they concluded that for the three compounds investigated, the rhesus monkey has skin penetration characteristics similar to those of man.

By the use of radiolabelled materials, Feldmann and Maibach (1970) investigated the skin penetration of 21 organic chemicals when applied to the forearms of human volunteers. The investigators found that the range for total absorption was greater than 250 times and that the difference in maximum absorption rate varied by more than 100 times. Continuing their human volunteer studies, Maibach *et al.* (1971) investigated the penetration of skin in different anatomical locations by using radiolabelled pesticides (parathion, malathion, and carbaryl), and their findings confirmed the observations of Marzulli (1962) that there were large differences in the penetrability of skin from different anatomical locations. In particular scrotal skin was found to be deficient in barrier properties. Feldmann and Maibach (1974) then went on to investigate the penetration of human skin by twelve pesticides and two of their findings were particularly relevant: (i) the carbamate insecticide carbaryl has exceptionally good skin penetrating properties, a fact that must be considered when carbaryl is being handled or used (Comer et al., 1975) and (ii) the quaternary herbicide diquat has virtually no skin penetrating ability, a fact that lends weight to the criticism made by McElligott (1972) of the use of the 24 hours' covered exposure in predictive acute toxicity testing.

Most chemicals are more toxic to the animal when exposure is by the oral route rather than where absorption is through the skin. There are some exceptions to this general rule. Shaffer and West (1960) showed that the acaricide tetram, administered as an aqueous solution, was more toxic to rats by the percutaneous route than when administered orally:

	LD_{50} (mg/kg) (95% confidence limits)	
	Oral	Percutaneous
Male	9 (7 to 13)	2 (1 to 3)
Female	8 (6 to 11)	2 (1 to 3)

Metcalf (1957) had shown that in aqueous solution tetram exists as an equilibrium mixture of salt and base, this may account for the absorption characteristics of the product.

$$
\left[\begin{array}{c} C_2H_5O \diagdown \diagup O \\ P \\ C_2H_5O \diagup \diagdown S.C_2H_4NH^+ \end{array} \begin{array}{c} C_2H_5 \\ | \\ \\ | \\ C_2H_5 \end{array} \right] \quad \begin{array}{c} COO^- \\ | \\ COOH \end{array}
$$

Tetram

Valuable human data having been obtained for several pesticides, Serat et al. (1975) have begun to apply mathematical models involving estimates of percutaneous toxicity for calculating suitable field re-entry intervals for agricultural workers.

Absorption through the eyes (perocular absorption)

The absorption of pesticides through the eyes is rarely a serious toxicological hazard because of the small surface area exposed and the efficiency of the protective mechanisms (i.e. blink reflex and tears). As long as the epithelium of the eyes remains intact it is impermeable to many molecules but provided that the toxicant has a suitable polar–non-polar balance penetration may occur (Swan and White, 1942; Kondritzer et al., 1959).

Holmstedt (1959) and Brown and Muir (1971) have reviewed perocular absorption of pesticides. More recently, Sinow and Wei (1973) have shown that the quaternary herbicide paraquat can be lethal to rabbits if applied directly to the surface of the eyes.

Absorption from the respiratory tract (inhalation exposure)

The respiratory tract provides an efficient absorptive surface for toxicants whether they be in the form of vapours, discrete particles (i.e. smokes and dusts), or atmosphere-borne droplets (i.e. aerosols and sprays). The respiratory tract is also receptive to aspirated vapours and fluids and this is a common cause of death when volatile pesticide formulations are ingested (Gerarde, 1963; Gerarde and Ahlstrom, 1966; Boyd, 1972). As a route for intoxication by pesticides inhalation is important (Oudbier et al., 1974) but it must be recognized that droplets and particles that are too large to pass into the respiratory tract may aggregate in the nasopharyngeal region and pass into the alimentary tract.

Meaningful predictive tests in inhalation toxicology are particularly difficult to perform (MacFarland, 1975) but there are many examples of attempts in the published literature (Niessen et al., 1963; Walker et al., 1972; Thorpe et al., 1972; Dean and Thorpe, 1972; Sachsse et al., 1973a and 1973b; Clark, 1973; Stevens et al., 1978). The range of techniques and equipment that may be used has been effectively reviewed by Drew and Laskin (1973).

There are published examples of human volunteer studies with inhaled pesticides. Dichlorvos, an organophosphorus insecticide active in the vapour phase, has been the subject of such investigations (Cavagna et al., 1969 and 1970; Cavagna and Vigliani, 1970) and Hartwell et al. (1964) similarly investigated the vapours of warmed parathion. Ganelin et al. (1964) even investigated the effects of parathion vapours on asthmatic subjects. Some definitive inhalation studies have been carried out under either real or simulated conditions of actual pesticide use, and the investigations have included different types of formulations such as sprays and dusts (Hartwell et al., 1964; Hartwell and Hayes, 1965; Wolfe et al., 1966 and 1967; Durham et al., 1972).

The use of the term 'acute' in inhalation toxicology requires special definition. Since an atmospheric dose must be expressible as a concentration and the physiological act of respiration is dynamic, it is not possible to allocate a specific dose intake to one occasion, therefore the acute toxicity must be expressed as a function of concentration in the atmosphere and time. Quite arbitrarily a time limit of 4 hours has been accepted by many toxicologists as the maximum time for an exposure to be described as being acute. Within limits, it has been shown that for some compounds the product of concentration and time to achieve the same response is constant:

$$CT = \text{constant}$$

when,

C = concentration of toxicant in atmosphere (mg m^{-3})

t = time (min)

The Ct = constant rule is generally attributed to Haber (1924). Bliss (1940) elaborated on Haber's rule and devised the formula:

$$\frac{[(CV_m) - D_e]tR}{W} = D$$

when,

D = dosage (mg/kg bodyweight) received during time t

C = concentration of toxicant (mg m^{-3})

V_m = minute volume rate or respiration (m^{-3} min)

D_e = detoxification rate (mg min^{-1})

t = time of exposure (min)

W = bodyweight (kg)

R = retention coefficient expressed as decimal fraction

However, MacFarland (1975) has suggested that a more realistic formula is:

$$\alpha = Ct \times M_v = \text{constant}$$

when,

α = retention (per cent)

M_v = minute volume for the exposed animal (ml min^{-1})

c = concentration of toxicant (mg m^{-3})

t = time of exposure in minutes

A convenient formula for calculating the retained dose in inhalation toxicology is:

$$\text{retained dose} = \frac{CtV_m\alpha}{W} \text{ mg/kg}$$

when,

C = concentration of toxicant in atmosphere (mg m^{-3})

t = duration of exposure (min)

V_m = volume of atmosphere respired (m^3 min^{-1})

α = fraction of inhaled dose retained

W = weight of subject (kg)

Sidorenko and Pinigin (1976) have attempted to apply acute inhalation toxicity data to predict more long-term effects by using the Ct principle.

Just as it is difficult to rationalize dosage for inhalation exposure because of the time factor, it is difficult to correlate the dosage with physiological parameters. Tenney and Remmers (1963) studied a large number of animals ranging in size from bats to whales and found that there exists a high degree of correlation between lung volume and bodyweight, between alveolar surface area and whole body oxygen consumption, and also between alveolar diameter and metabolic rate per unit of bodyweight. (N.B. When plotted on log–log scale the correlation coefficients for these three were 1.02, 1.00, and -0.71, respectively, and for each of the plots 21 animal species were included.)

It is possible to define deposition of particulate materials in the respiratory tract (Greene, 1971; Hicks, 1975), but calculations and deductions are generally based on the assumption that all particles are uniform in shape, and this assumption is often incorrect. Other reviews of the physical, mathematical, and physiological implications of particulates and aerosols in relation to the respiratory tract have been provided by Morrow (1960), Hatch and Gross (1964), and by Mercer (1973). Morrow (1960) tabulated the major factors involved when particulate matter affects the respiratory tract and the result is reproduced here as Table 5.2.

As with other organs, the lungs are capable of metabolic activity and the lungs of different species vary in their capability to metabolize toxicants (Brown, E. A. B., 1974). The permeability of the lung mucosa varies for different toxicants in various species. Mitchell and Schanker (1973) found that the mouse lung pulmonary membrane was more permeable than that of the rat lung for several organic chemicals. Burton *et al.* (1974) studied the uptake of four herbicides (2,4-D; 2,4,5-T; aminotriazole, and diquat) from the lungs of rats and then compared the absorption rates with concentrations, molecular weights, and lipid solubilities; they concluded that with this small series absorption occurred by simple diffusion across a lipid–pore-type membrane.

2,4-D   2,4,5-T   Aminotriazole

Table 5.2 Major factors involved in the respiratory toxicology of particulate matter (after Morrow, 1960)

Factors	Particles involved	Related factors	Primary factors	Special considerations
Sedimentation	>0.1 μm to <50 μm	Particle shape and density Particulate concentration (aggregation), 'slip', hygroscopicity.	To cause dust deposition in nasal pharynx and tracheal-bronchial tree.	Highly significant in toxicological studies, probably the most important deposition factors. Especially significant with 'soluble or absorbable' dusts.
Inertia	<50 μm	Same as above plus relative velocities of particle and air.	Same as above with tendency to promote earlier deposition.	
Brownian motion	>0.002 μm to <0.5 μm	Electric charge, hygroscopicity, particle concentration (aggregation), thermal gradients.	Dust deposition where large and intimate surfaces involved, viz. lung bronchioles and parenchyma.	Most important when dust is insoluble and sub-micronic. Also significant when these dusts serve as vectors.
Respiratory frequency	All sizes	Air velocities, residence times, turbulence, dead space ventilation.	Increasing tends to decrease deposition (possibly very high rates, e.g. >20 may increase deposition).	Exercise, physical labour, and heated environs will have variable effects on subjects but, in general, will tend to increase both these factors together.
Tidal volume	All sizes	Number of particles, alveolar ventilation, residence time.	Increasing tends to increase deposition (even at constant minute volume).	

In a detailed study with more than 400 vapours, Ljublina and Rabotnikova (1970) and Ljublina and Filov (1975) were able to make toxicity predictions from the known physico-chemical properties of each compound. These investigations may be considered as being complementary to the work of Ferguson (1939) and Hansch (1970) and similar to the objectives of Enslein et al. (1977).

Some toxicants are better absorbed from the respiratory tract than from the alimentary tract. Hwang and Schanker (1974) demonstrated that the insecticidal carbamate carbaryl is absorbed 2.5 times faster from the respiratory tract of the rat than it is from the alimentary tract in the same species. From the respiratory tract it was found, by accident, that man could absorb sufficient of the organophosphorus compound malathion to be lethal (Sellassie and Lester, 1971). Using a technique by which aerosols of radiolabelled carbaryl, leptophos, parathion, and chlordane were placed directly into the trachea, Nye and Dorough (1976) found that the ultimate fate of each pesticide did not differ from that resulting from exposure by the oral route.

Some fluoro-compounds are used as propellants for pesticidal aerosols and some of these propellants have been found to be capable of causing a sensitization of the heart to stress (Clayton, 1967; Taylor and Harris, 1970; Harris, 1973; Aviado, 1975); however, for environmental as well as toxicological reasons, the use of these propellants has diminished.

Absorption from other routes (parenteral exposure)

Because of the influence of route of administration on the efficacy of therapeutic agents, it is common in bio-pharmaceutics to utilize parenteral routes of exposure (Dollery et al., 1971; Rowland, 1972). In predictive acute toxicity testing with pesticides the use of parenteral routes can be helpful in assessing metabolic effects rather than acting as a direct measure of hazard.

When some chemicals are injected into the peritoneal cavity efficient absorption can occur (Kruger et al., 1962) and by means of radiolabelled compounds it has been shown that toxicants administered intraperitoneally are primarily absorbed through the portal circulation and thence pass through the liver before reaching other organs (Lukas et al., 1971). However, the rate at which a compound is delivered to the liver, whether from the alimentary canal or from the intraperitoneal route, can influence the amount of the administered dose that reaches other targets and this rate is more complex than a straightforward Michaelis–Menten kinetic process would predict (Riegelman and Rowland, 1974).

Working with several organophosphorus pesticides, Natoff (1967) demonstrated the relative importance of liver metabolism in their acute toxicity. Natoff administered compounds by the oral and intraperitoneal routes to involve the liver (i.e. 'hepatic routes') and by subcutaneous and intravenous injection (i.e. 'peripheral routes'), and made judgements as to the influence of hepatic metabolism on the toxicants. Although this simple approach has merit for preliminary metabolic screening, some caution is required before the results are interpreted for, although the liver may be the primary route for metabolism of many compounds, metabolic conversion by other routes may be operative. An example of this alternative route metabolism has been shown to occur with the conversion of parathion *in vivo* into paraoxon when the liver has been interfered with either chemically or surgically (Alary and Brodeur, 1969 and 1970; Neal, 1972; Jacobsen *et al.*, 1973).

Although Natoff (1967) described the subcutaneous route as a means of achieving the 'peripheral route', subcutaneous injection is not often used in predictive toxicology with pesticides. The absorption kinetics for chemicals from the subcutaneous route have been fully investigated because of the importance of this route of administration in bio-pharmaceutics (Ballard and Menczel, 1967; Secher-Hansen *et al.*, 1967a and 1967b).

The intravenous route has been used in the investigation of several pesticides. Walsh and Fink (1972) used the route to study the bio-distribution of the chlorinated hydrocarbon insecticides endrin and dieldrin in mice, and Verschoyle and Barnes (1972) and Barnes and Verschoyle (1974) studied the synthetic pyrethroids in this way. Certainly the distribution of toxicant within the body is affected by the route of administration as well as by the metabolism of the toxicant (Riegelman and Rowland, 1974). Heath and Vandekar (1957), Vandekar and Heath (1957), and Vandekar (1958) found that the pesticide demeton-methyl undergoes alkylation when stored or when diluted with water, the alkylsulphonium product that is formed has an acute oral toxicity in the rat that is almost identical to that of demeton-methyl but by intravenous injection in the rat, the alkylsulphonium compound increases the toxicity of the pesticide by between 40 and 100 times.

The influence of the bio-distribution is particularly apparent with some compounds injected intravenously. Freedman and Himwich (1949) injected di-isopropyl fluorophosphate (DFP) into rabbits using venous routes, both the femoral and the portal veins, and also arterial routes using both the femoral and the carotid arteries. Freedman and Himwich obtained very different LD_{50} values (summarized in Table 5.3) and very different influences on the brain cholinesterases. The rate of injection of toxicants by the intravenous route can be critical to the acute toxicity values obtained.

Intracerebral injection has been used by some investigators to assess the effects of organophosphorus compounds in brain cholinesterases without the intervening effects of liver metabolism and the blood-brain barrier (Rainsford, 1978).

Nabb *et al.* (1966) found that parathion was only 10 times less toxic than

Table 5.3 Data on the acute toxicity of di-isopropyl fluorophosphate (DFP) administered to rabbits by different routes.
(Data from Freedman and Himwich, 1949)

Route	LD_{50} mg/kg ± S.E.	Ratio*
Both carotid arteries	0.109 ± 0.030	1
One carotid artery	0.456 ± 0.061	4
Femoral vein	0.478 ± 0.063	4
Femoral artery	0.858 ± 0.082	8
Portal vein	2.30 ± 0.15	22

*Value for administration via both carotid arteries arbitrarily taken
as 1.

paraoxon when administered intravenously to rabbits but when applied to
the skin parathion was 55 times less toxic than paraoxon. Much of this
difference was accounted for by the large difference in skin penetrating
ability of the two compounds.

Compound	Rate of uptake via the skin
Parathion	$0.059 \ \mu g \min^{-1} cm^{-2}$
Paraoxon	$0.32 \ \ \mu g \min^{-1} cm^{-2}$

CHAPTER 6

The acute toxicology of pesticides in perspective

The historical development and the projected future requirements for pesticides indicate that there will be a continuing demand for pesticides but that the rate of innovation may have plateaued. However, for as long as pesticides are used it is inevitable that there will be associated incidents of acute intoxication involving non-target species.

Because of the increasing demands for pesticides and other commercial pressures, syntheses are sometimes varied and the pesticide that is made available may not accord with the specification of the product used in the predictive acute toxicity tests. The pesticide used may contain aberrant impurities and sometimes these may be disastrously toxic; this is exemplified by the occurrence of 2,3,7,8-tetrachlorobenzo-p-dioxin in the herbicide 2,3,4-T and by the formation of isomalathion in malathion formulations stored under adverse conditions and used for malaria eradication in Pakistan (Umetsu *et al.*, 1977; Baker Jr. *et al.*, 1978).

Episodes of acute intoxication involving humans will *a priori* continue to be biased towards the less socially advanced populations although incidents of acute intoxication due to accidents during manufacturing, handling, formulating, and transportation will continue to affect a wider spectrum of people. Acute intoxication due to human folly transcends social and intellectual boundries.

Acute intoxication of vertebrate species other than man will inevitably occur but by the development of responsible attitudes these incidents could be substantially diminished. Attitudes towards the protection of natural and domesticated fauna from intoxication by pesticides are not always paramount in the minds of all people.

With the acute toxicity of pesticides the experimental toxicologist is presented with a dilemma (i.e. a choice between alternatives that appear to be equally undesirable). If no predictive acute toxicity tests were carried out, then there would not be any information on which to base assessment of hazard. The alternative is that predictive tests are performed in the light of current knowledge and the toxicologist is faced with the problem of interpreting data by an extrapolative process that is essentially unique for each pesticide. Too often toxicologists and others responsible for utilizing the information approach the subject of acute toxicity on the assumption that there are simple rules governing the interpretation of experimental data in terms of hazard assessment, whereas the critical analysis presented in this monograph clearly shows that this is not the case.

In both experimental predictive toxicology and in the real hazard situation, the route of exposure to the toxicant can be of fundamental importance. Many pesticides are highly toxic to non-target species, but, in practice, are reasonably safe because they are not presented in a way that allows absorption into the animal. It is not solely the fact that absorption occurs but rather the rate of absorption that is critical in relation to the overall pharmacokinetics that manifests an acute toxic response. The major routes in man for system effects due to adventitious pesticide exposure are in descending order of likelihood, skin, ingestion, inhalation and, rarely, the eyes and parenteral routes. With vertebrate species other than man, ingestion is likely to be the prime cause of intoxication. Deliberate exposure of humans to pesticides is likely to be by ingestion but the other routes of exposure are not entirely precluded.

Adventitious exposure of people to pesticides is not restricted to personnel engaged in agricultural and horticultural activities. There are also many people associated with manufacturing, formulating, transporting, and otherwise handling pesticides as well as the general public who may be affected by such things as pesticide spray drift. Carelessness in handling, packaging, and transporting pesticides can affect the safety of people and other animals not knowingly associated with the pesticides.

The improper use of pesticides can represent a significant threat to non-target species. Ancillary incidents such as fires and explosions can exaggerate the incidence of acute intoxications associated with the manufacturing and handling of pesticides by increasing the distribution of the pesticide into the environment or by the formation of toxic products of pyrolysis.

The ranking of hazard for chemicals is not easy (Jones, 1978) and acute toxicity is only one of the many factors to be considered. If it is accepted that acute toxicity tests are necessary then the use of the common routes of exposure experienced in the hazard situation (i.e. oral, percutaneous, and inhalation routes) is sensible. The use of parenteral routes for exposure in investigative toxicology can be justified on the basis that useful data on the metabolism of the compound can be obtained easily; however, it is more difficult to rationalize the need for LD_{50} values obtained by parenteral administration as part of the obligatory acute toxicity data required for pesticide registration in some countries because there is non-discriminatory legislation in those countries covering all types of chemicals.

Parenteral administration of toxicants can give rise to irrelevant findings due to physico-chemical effects such as the influence of osmolarity, volume (e.g hypervolaemia following intravenous injection), or pH. Irritant chemicals may cause peritonitis if administered by the intraperitoneal route.

It is a practical necessity that most acute toxicity tests are carried out using species that are not in fact the subject of most, or even any, concern. The extensive use of the laboratory rat (*Rattus norvegicus*) and the laboratory mouse (*Mus musculus*) for acute toxicity tests illustrates this point. Many tests are performed in order to assess hazard to man but, although man is an accessible species, there are moral, legal, and practical difficulties associated with the use of man as a test species. It is easier to carry out tests aimed at defining hazard to non-human species in more closely related animals; however, there are still many pitfalls associated with the use of non-feral species for predicting effects on wildlife and also there are often significant differences between the responses observed in apparently closely related animals.

The information obtained from experiments, on the acute toxicity of products is generally expressed in terms of quantity of toxicant per unit of bodyweight or, less often, as quantity of toxicant per unit of body surface-area. Neither of the variables associated with the test animal (i.e. bodyweight or body surface-area) is entirely a logical function to use. Some form of age-linked metabolic bodyweight could be considered as a better species variable, but even if that were possible, there are theoretical objections to its use. On the basis of the very large amount of information available on the toxicity of numerous chemicals to many different species, it is probable that the use of quantity of toxicant per unit of bodyweight is an appropriate expression of the results for at least 80% of the pesticides that have been tested for acute toxicity to laboratory animals. The proviso must be added that this dose–bodyweight relationship applies only to data generated in adult animals; there is no simple correlation between age and susceptibility to intoxication, and neo-natal and young animals may well respond to intoxication in a way that is different from that in adults.

Among the approximately 20% of pesticides for which the dose–bodyweight relationship is inappropriate are those products that are toxic to vertebrates because of effects on basal metabolism. The acute toxicities of these are more likely to be quantitatively expressable as quantity of toxicant per unit of body surface-area or, occasionally, as quantity of toxicant per animal.

The sex of the exposed animal can influence the response to intoxication by pesticides; however, the differences in response are generally quantitative rather than qualitative. Of all the species that have been used for acute toxicity testing, the infleunce of sex on response to toxicants is generally greatest in rodents and is sometimes only apparent in the laboratory rat although this observation may be biased because more rats have used for the investigation of pesticides than any other species. When sex differences in response have been observed in more than one species, the sex ratios are very often quite different in each species and may even be reversed in quite closely related species. Sex differences in response are related to differences in the intrinsic pharmacokinetics of the pesticide in animals of each sex and to the species. Large sex differences in susceptibility to intoxication, and neo-natal and young animals may well in laboratory rats; in the majority of cases the females are more susceptible than the males but there are several examples in which the reverse is true. The sex differences in response to toxicants are often accentuated if the exposure is through the skin.

Socio-economic and other demographic factors have profoundly influenced the distribution of pesticide intoxication in man. Unlike the subject of susceptibility of drugs, there has been little rigorous study of ethnic factors in the intrinsic response to acute intoxication by pesticides. There are numerous examples in which the differences in strain or breed of animals have given rise to differences in susceptibility to intoxication by pesticides and these differences may be due to differences in distribution and metabolism of the toxicant; therefore it is expected that similar ethnic variation will occur in man.

Although biorhythms and stress are well-known phenomena in man there is little unequivocal information to support the idea that they affect the response of man to pesticides. It is possible that the more subtle acute effects of intoxication may be exacerbated and this could affect the performance of exposed personnel (e.g. the influence of an organophosphorus insecticide on the pilot of an aircraft engaged in crop spraying might adversely affect the pilot's acuity with consequential effects). Stress and biorhythms are much more apparent in many animals other than man and they can be readily induced and manipulated under experimental conditions. Generally the effects of stress in animals have not been found to be great in relation to the intrinsic acute response but in the wildlife situation the indirect effects of stress, such as increased susceptibility to predation, may be more important.

The relationship between ambient temperature and humidity and the toxic effects of pesticides in vertebrate animals is not linear. Depending on the toxicant the relationship between ambient temperature and toxic response may be large or may be negligible; if it is not negligible the response may be either positive or negative (i.e. an increase in ambient temperature may raise or lower the lethal or effect dose, and the converse). For man there is an increased risk in hot climates, not because of an increased intrinsic toxicity, but because of a disinclination or a frank inability to use adequate protective equipment. There are some pesticides that may affect body temperature (e.g. DNOC) but the more subtle effects of chemicals on the thermoregulatory function (e.g. some organophosphates) are probably inconsequential, in relation to their other toxic properties, except perhaps in small animals. Poikilothermal animals do not behave in a consistent way under the influence of pesticides under different conditions of ambient temperature.

Innovators of new pesticides endeavour to achieve a high target specificity and this clearly includes attempting to achieve a potent pesticidal action with a minimum toxicity to non-target vertebrates. In the case of the rodenticides and some avicides the objective is toxicity to vermin with minimum toxicity to other vertebrates. On occasions highly toxic insecticides are deliberately used to kill vertebrate pests and this practice is not without danger.

Because of the complexity of the vertebrate animals and the variability of pesticides associated with those organisms, it is not possible to develop a teleological argument relating susceptibility to pesticide intoxication with phylogenetic characteristics. There is no evidence that the primates are necessarily better indicators of acute intoxication by pesticides in man than are laboratory rodents. There is no consistent pattern that allows the assumption that relative susceptibility will be in the order: fish, amphibians, reptiles, birds, mammals, or the reverse order, although this might have been an attractive hypothesis on the basis of evolutionary trends.

Since the term 'acute' is imprecise and only conveys the meaning 'of short duration', it has been necessary to establish conventions in relation to time as a function. Exposures involving toxicants in the environment need a more defined time function in order to quantify toxicity than do exposures in which the subject receives a dose of toxicant by other routes. Accepting the convention that the term acute is related to the exposure than the response to intoxication may be delayed or slow as was found with the response of animals to 2,3,7,8-tetrachlorobenzo-p-dioxin (i.e. slow death due to progressive hepatotoxicity followed a single acute exposure) or the delayed neurotoxicity associated with acute exposure of some organophosphorus compounds.

The scientific value of necropsies carried out on dead animals from predictive acute toxicity tests is often debated. In many cases *post-mortem* examination is wasted effort, especially in the case of animals that have died rapidly following exposure to the toxicant; however, necropsies should be performed on animals that exhibit delayed or prolonged signs of intoxication or that die several days after dosing.

Formulation can profoundly affect the efficacy of pesticides and also increase or decrease their acute toxicities to non-target species and this has major implications in relation to safety. The influence on safety may be brought about in several ways; the vehicle may influence absorption by increasing or decreasing uptake into the animal and this is further influenced by the route of exposure. Alternatively, the formulated pesticides may be so diluted that the total amount of formulation that would have to be assimilated to achieve a toxic effect would be large and hence self-limiting, although the toxic dose in terms of active pesticide may still appear to be small. Formulation of pesticides can be critical in terms of toxicity to all non-target species. Bait formulation can be attractive to animals other than those intended to be tempted to ingest them. Dressed seed is attractive to some birds and this has been the cause of many bird deaths. There is a critical balance between spray droplet characteristics that will be effective against the pests and spray drift away from intended target areas that may cause adventitious exposure in non-target species. The influence of formulation on potential hazard is great and for this reason the acute toxicity of a pesticide formulation should always be assessed in addition to any investigations carried out on the technical pesticide as such.

Theoretically there should be a lower limit to the amount of a toxicant that may produce an acute intoxication. It is probable that the most acutely toxic chemical that has been associated with pesticides on a large scale has been 2,3,7,8-tetrachlorobenzo-p-dioxin, a contaminant of some batches of the herbicide 2,4,5-T and also an environmental contaminant associated with the manufacture of the trichlorophenols used as intermediates in the synthesis of several pesticides. This particular dioxin has an acute oral LD_{50} value that is measurable in micrograms per kilogram bodyweight. Of all the pesticides internationally approved for use, only one has an oral LD_{50} value, in the rat, of less than 1 mg/kg, that is the carbamate insecticide aldicarb. There are, of course, some very toxic chemicals not associated with pesticidal use, some of the most potent of these are naturally occurring toxins.

Some pesticides have low percutaneous toxicities although they are highly toxic if ingested, this is important as the skin is the most likely route of accidental exposure. In practice the ease with which acute intoxication can be reversed by the use of antidotes can be critical; for some pesticides there are no specific antidotes and for some other metabolic activation or lethal synthesis may complicate the efficacy of antidotal therapy.

Exposure to more than one pesticide or even repeated exposure to the same pesticide can affect the acute response. The overall effect can be additive, greater than or less than additive and the response may be influenced by the time sequence of the multiple exposures. Although there are possibilities of dangerous toxic interactions, there is little real evidence of serious consequences having occurred from multiple exposures to pesticides in use. The possibility of man or other animals being exposed to pesticides and then either simultaneously or subsequently exposed to other chemicals, such as therapeutic agents, must be construed as a potential hazard, but there is little evidence that this has been a clinical problem.

The experimental assessment of acute toxicity is most often linked to population effects. For statistical purposes the greatest amount of interest is generally centred on results involving 50% of the exposed population and this has provided a convenient quantification, the LD_{50} value, for use in toxicology. It would be more useful to be able to obtain meaningful data on effects involving much smaller fractions that half of the exposed population and the importance of the response in the individual can be as important as a population effect. Great care must be exercised in the extrapolation of data from experiments designed to assess the LD_{50} value in order to assess smaller percentage effects.

E

In conclusion it must be stated that although the derivation of information on acute toxicity by the use of animal model followed by a process of extrapolation is imperfect, there is no indication that techniques utilizing non-sentient organisms or other *in vitro* techniques will provide as much meaningful information as that achieved by the use of animals. Guarded optimism that the use of a data bank, associated with modern computer techniques, could aid predictive acute toxicology is permissible, but the investment in setting up a meaningful facility would be enormous and it is axiomatic that the undertaking of such a project could only be meaningful if the data to be included were impeccable and this, in its turn, would necessitate a professional audit of all data intended for inclusion.

Despite the attitudes of some regulatory authorities, it is not sensible to attribute too much meaning to the LD_{50} value, nor to assign a minimum value for the LD_{50} below which a pesticide would be acceptable for use. There are sub-lethal and irreversible effects that may be highly undesirable but may be associated with compounds with high LD_{50} values. Acute toxicology is not concerned solely with lethality but also with sub-lethal toxic effects and in this respect one must agree, at least in part, with the statement attributed to the late Lord Platt, that 'The LD_{50} is most extravagant in the use of animals; it is questionable whether it is morally or ethically sound in most cases and whether it gives the results we want to answer the question we need to put'. The determination of an LD_{50} value with reasonable precision but associated with a more comprehensive assessment of other effects following acute exposure must form part of the detailed risk–benefit analysis associated with the development of any pesticide. The risk–benefit analysis must include the potential hazard to man and other vertebrates associated with the pesticide during its synthesis, formulation, transportation, use, and disposal as well as its value as a pesticide, and in the state of current knowledge there is a need for predictive acute toxicity tests in order to make any sort of hazard assessment.

References

Abou-Donia, M. B., Othman, M. A., Tantawy, G., Khalil, A. Z. and Shawer, M. F. (1974). Neurotoxic effect of leptophos. *Experientia*, **30**, 63–64.

Abou-el-Makarem, M. M., Millburn, P., Smith, R. L. and Williams, R. T. (1967). Biliary excretion of foreign compounds: Species differences in biliary excretion. *Biochem. J.*, **105**, 1289–1293.

Adamson, R. H. (1967). Drug metabolism in marine vertebrates. *Fed. Proc.*, **26**, 1047–1055.

Adolph, E. F. (1949). Quantitative relations in the physiological constitutions of mammals. *Science*, **109**, 579–585.

Agthe, C., Garcia, H., Schubik, P., Tomatis, L. and Wenyon, E. (1970). Study on the potential carcinogenicity of DDT in the Syrian golden hamster. *Proc. Soc. Exptl Biol. Med.*, **134**, 113–116.

Ahdaya, S. M., Shah, P. V. and Guthrie, F. E. (1976). Thermoregulation in mice treated with parathion, carbaryl or DDT. *Tox. Appl. Pharmacol.*, **35**, 575–580.

Ahdaya, S. M., Shah, P. V. and Guthrie, F. E. (1978). Comparative penetration (*in vivo*) of insecticides through the skin and gastrointestinal tract of mice. 17th Annual Meeting Society of Toxicology (San Francisco—March 1978) Abstract only.

Alabaster, J. S. (1969a). Survival of fish in 164 herbicides, insecticides, fungicides, wetting agents and miscellaneous substances. *Int. Pest Control*, **11**, 29–35.

Alabaster, J. S. (1969b). Evaluating risks of pesticides to fish. *Proc. 5th Br. Insectic. Fungic. Conf.* (Brighton—England).

Alary, J. G. and Brodeur, J. (1969). Studies on the mechanism of phenobarbital-induced protection against parathion in adult female rats. *J. Pharmacol. exptl Ther.*, **169**, 159–167.

Alary, J. G. and Brodeur, J. (1970). Correlation between the activity of liver enzymes and the LD_{50} of parathion in the rat. *Canad. J. Physiol. Pharmacol.*, **48**, 829–831.

Albert, J. R. and Stearns, S. M. (1974). Delayed neurotoxic potential of a series of alkyl esters of 2,2,dichlorovinyl phosphoric acid in the chicken. *Tox. Appl. Pharmacol.*, **29**, 136.

Albert, J. R., Stearns, S. M. and Flick, S. C. (1974). Drug interaction studies in the cat: Vapona insecticide flea collars. *Feline Practice* (Jan.–Feb.) 43–47.

Albornoz, A. L. (1973). Statistical study of the first year's activity of the Caracas Poison Control Centre. (in French). *Bull. Med. Leg. Toxicol.*, **16**, 149–150.

Alcock, S. J. (1971). An anti-inflammatory compound: Non-toxic to animals but with an adverse action in man. *Proc. Europ. Soc. Study of Drug Tox.*, **12**, 184–190.

Aldridge, W. N., Barnes, J. M. and Johnson, M. K. (1969). Studies on delayed neurotoxicity produced by some organophosphorus compounds in, 'Biological effects of Pesticides in Mammalian Systems'. *Ann. N.Y. Acad. Sci.*, **160**, 314–322.

Allcroft, R. and Jones J. S. L. (1969). Fluoroacetamide poisoning: 1. Toxicity in dairy cattle; clinical history and preliminary investigations. *Vet. Rec.*, **84**, 399–402.

Allcroft, R., Salt, F. J., Peters, R. A. and Shorthouse, M. (1969). Fluoroacetamide poisoning: 2. Toxicity in dairy cattle; confirmation of diagnosis. *Vet. Rec.*, **84**, 403–408.

Allen, S. D., van Kampen, K. R. and Brooks, D. R. (1978). Evaluation of the feline dichlorvos (DDVP) flea collar. *Feline Practice*, **8**, 9–16.

Allmark, M. G. (1951). A collaborative study on the acute toxicity testing of several drugs. *J. Am. Pharm. Assoc.*, **40**, 27–31.

Amarasingahm, R. D. and Ti Thiow Hee (1976). A review of poisoning cases examined by the Department of Chemistry, Malaysia from 1968–1972. *Med. J. Malaysia*, **30**, 185–193.

Amure, J. and Stuart, J. C. (1978). Dieldrin toxicity in poultry associated with wood shavings. *Vet. Rec.*, **102**, 387 only.

Anderson, L. S., Warner, D. L., Parker, J. E., Bluman, N. and Page, B. D. (1965). Parathion poisoning from flannelette sheets. *Canad. Med. Ass. J.*, **92**, 809–813.

Anderson, P. D. and Weber, L. J. (1975). Toxic response as a quantitative function of body-size. *Tox. Appl. Pharmacol.*, **33**, 471–483.

121

E*

122

Ando, H. Y., Ho, N. F. H. and Higuchi, W. I. (1977). Skin as an active metabolizing barrier. 1. Theoretical analysis of topical bioavailability. *J. Pharm. Sci.*, **66**, 1525–1528.

Angel, G. (1969). Starvation, stress and the blood–brain barrier. *Dis. Nerv. Syst.*, **30**, 94–97.

Angelakos, E. T. (1960). Lack of relationship between bodyweight and pharmacological effect exemplified by histamine toxicity in mice. *Proc. Soc. exptl Biol. Med.*, **103**, 296–298.

Arnan, A. (1971). Experience in the WHO field programme for evaluating the safety of new insecticides. *Bull. Wld Hlth Org.*, **44**, 274–276.

Arterberry, J. D., Bonicaci, R. W., Nash, E. W. and Quinby, G. E. (1962). Potentiation of phosphorus insecticides by phenothiazine derivatives. Possible hazard with report of a fatal case. *J. Amer. Med. Assoc.*, **182**, 848–850.

Arthur, B. W. and Casida, J. E. (1957). Metabolism and selectivity of *o,o*-dimethyl 2,2,2,-trichloro-1-hydroxyethyl phosphonate and its acetyl and vinyl derivatives. *J. Agr. Food Chem.*, **5**, 186–192.

Aschheim, E. (1965). Kinetic characterization of the terminal vascular bed during inflammation. *Am. J. Physiol.*, **208**, 270–274.

Ashford, J. R. (1959). An approach to the analysis of data for semi-quantal responses in biological assay. *Biometrics*, **15**, 573–581.

Aston, R. A., Sekino, E. and Greifenstein, F. E. (1962). Quantitation of drug effects upon conditioned avoidance behaviour in rats. *Toxicol. Appl. Pharmacol.*, **4**, 393–401.

Atabaev, S. T. and Kur, D. A. (1978). Effect of pesticides on energy metabolism under high temperature conditions (in Russian). *Gig. Sanit.*, **43**, 32–36. (*Pestic. Abs.* 78–1862).

Atzert, S. P. (1971). A review of sodium monofluoroacetate (compound 1080) its properties, toxicology and use in predator and rodent control. *U.S. Dept. of the Interior (Fish and Wildlife Service): Special Scientific Report—Wildlife No. 146.*

Aviado, D. M. (1975). Toxicity of aerosols. *J. Clin. Pharmacol.*, **15**, 86–104.

Ayres, J. W. and Laskar, P. A. (1974). Evaluation of mathematical models for diffusion from semi-solids. *J. Pharm. Sci.*, **63**, 351–356.

Baba, K., Nara, M., Iwahashi, Y., Sasaki, T. and Ohsuga, H. (1976). Toxicity of pesticides to marine fish (in Japanese). *Shizuoka-ken Suisan Shikengo Jigyo Hokoku*—80–83.

Baer, H. (1971). Long-term isolation stress and its effects on drug response in rodents. *Lab. Anim. Sci.*, **21**, 341–349.

Baetjer, A. M. and Smith, R. (1956). Effect of environmental temperature on reaction of mice to parathion, an anticholinesterase agent. *Am. J. Physiol.*, **186**, 39–46.

Baker, Jr, E. L., Warren, M., Zack, M., Dobbin, R. D., Miles, J. W., Miller, J., Alderman, L., Teeters, W. R. (1978). Epidemic malathion poisoning in Pakistan malaria workers. *Lancet*, **i**, 31–34.

Ball, W. L., Sinclair, J. W., Crevier, M. and Kay, K. (1954). Modifications of parathion's toxicity for rats by pretreatment with chlorinated hydrocarbon insecticides. *Can. J. Biochem. Physiol.*, **32**, 440–445.

Ballard, B. E. and Menczel, E. (1967). Subcutaneous absorption kinetics of benzyl alcohol. *J. Pharm. Sci.*, **56**, 1476–1485.

Balogh, K. and Merk, F. B. (1973). Ultrastructure of renal collecting tubules following ingestion of a bipyridinium herbicide (Morfamquat). *Experientia*, **29**, 1101–1103.

Barlow, J. N. (1977). 'Toxicology and safety evaluation of Phosvel to Egyptian water buffalo' in, *Pesticide Management and Insecticide Resistance*. Editors: D. L. Watson and A. W. A. Brown. Academic Press—N.Y., San Francisco, and London.

Barnes, J. M. (1953). *Toxic Hazards of Certain Pesticides to Man*. World Health Organisation—Geneva.

Barnes, J. M. (1963). Toxic hazards from drugs. *J. Pharm. Pharmacol.*, **15**, 75T–91T.

Barnes, J. M. (1973). Toxicology of agricultural chemicals. *Outlook on Agriculture*, **7**, 97–101.

Barnes, J. M. (1974). 'Anticholinesterases: Some problems in understanding their effects in whole animals' in, *Forensic Toxicology*. Editor: B. Ballantyne. John Wright and Sons, Ltd.—Bristol.

Barnes, J. M. and Verschoyle, R. D. (1974). Toxicity of new pyrethroid insecticides. *Nature*, **248**, 711.

Barr, W. H. (1969). Factors involved in the assessment of systemic or biologic availability of drug products. *Drug Info. Bull.*, **3**, 27–45.

Barrer, R. M. (1941). *Diffusion in and through Solids*. Cambridge University Press—Cambridge.

Bartek, M. J., Labudde, J. A. and Maibach, H. I. (1972). Skin permeability *in vivo*: Comparison in rat, rabbit, pig, and man. *J. Invest. Derm.*, **58**, 114–123.

123

Bartsch, W., Sponer, G., Dietmann, K. and Fuchs, G. (1976). Acute toxicity of various solvents in the mouse and rat. *Arzneim.——Forsch*, **26**, 1581–1583.

Bass, S. W., Triolo, A. J. and Coon, J. M. (1972). Effect of DDT on the toxicity and metabolism of parathion in mice. *Toxicol. Appl. Pharmacol.*, **22**, 684–693.

Basu, T. K. and Dickerson, J. W. T. (1974). Inter-relationships of nutrition and the metabolism of drugs. *Chem. Biol. Interactions*, **8**, 193–206.

Bathe, R., Sachsse, K., Ullman, L., Hörmann, W. D., Zak, F. and Hess, R. (1974). The evaluation of fish toxicity in the laboratory. *Proc. 16th Meeting European Society for the Study of Drug Toxicity* (Carlsbad—CSSR).

Bathe, R., Ullman, L., Sachsse, K. and Hess, R. (1976). Relationship between toxicity to fish and to mammals: A comparative study under defined laboratory conditions. *Proc. Europ. Soc. Toxicol.*, **17**, 351–355.

Becker, W. A. (1962). Choice of animals and sensitivity of experiments. *Nature*, **193**, 1264–1266.

Beckett, A. H. and Hossie, R. D. (1971). 'Buccal absorption of drugs' in, *Handbook of Experimental Pharmacology*, Vol. 28 (Pt. 1). Editors: B. B. Brodie and J. R. Gillette, Springer-Verlag—Berlin, Heidelberg and N.Y.

Bedford, C. T. and Hutson, D. H. (1976). The comparative metabolism in rodents of the isomeric insecticides dieldrin and endrin. *Chem. Ind.*, Issue No. 110, 440–447.

Bedford, C. T., Hutson, D. H. and Natoff, I. L. (1975). The acute toxicity of endrin and its metabolites to rats. *Tox. Appl. Pharmacol.*, **33**, 115–121.

Bein, H. J. (1963). Rational and irrational numbers in toxicology. *Proc. Europ. Soc. Study of Drug Toxicity*, **2**, 15–26.

Belehrádek, J. (1957). A unified theory of cellular rate processes based upon an analysis of temperature action. *Protoplasma*, **48**, 53–71.

Bell, A., Barnes, R. and Simpson, G. R. (1968). Cases of absorption and poisoning by the pesticide Phosdrin. *Med. J. Austr.*, **1**, 178–180.

Bell, J. (1972). The acute toxicity of four common poisons to the opossum. *N.Z. Vet. J.*, **20**, 212–214.

Bellet, E. M. and Casida, J. E. (1973). Bicyclic phosphorus esters: high toxicity without cholinesterase inhibition. *Science*, **182**, 1135–1136.

Ben, M., Dixon, R. L., Adamson, R. H., Feinman, H. and Rall, D. P. (1964). Toxicity of various drugs using dimethyl sulphoxide as a solvent. *Pharmacologist*, **6**, 189.

Benjamin, B. and Haycocks, H. W. (1970). *The Analysis of Mortality and Other Actuarial Statistics*. Cambridge University Press—Cambridge.

Benke, G. M. and Murphy, S. D. (1975). The influence of age on the toxicity and metabolism of methyl parathion and parathion in male and female rats. *Tox. Appl. Pharmacol.*, **31**, 254–269.

Benke, G. M., Cheever, K. L., Mirer, F. E. and Murphy, S. D. (1974). Comparative toxicity, anticholinesterase action and metabolism of methyl parathion and parathion in sunfish and mice. *Tox. Appl. Pharmacol.*, **28**, 97–109.

Bennett, D. (1972). Accidental poisoning in a retriever puppy by a new rodenticide. *Vet. Rec.*, **91**, 609–610.

Benson, W. W. (1973). The pesticide fire: A potential killer. *Fire Command* (February) 1–3.

Berkson, J. (1944). Application of the logistic function to bio-assay. *J. Amer. Statist. Assoc.*, **39**, 357–365.

Beroza, M., Inscoe, M. N., Schwartz, P. H., Keplinger, M. L. and Mastri, C. W. (1975). Acute toxicity studies with insect attractants. *Tox. Appl. Pharmacol.*, **31**, 421–429.

Bidstrup, P. L., Bonnell, J. A. L. and Harvey, D. G. (1952). Prevention of acute dinitro-orthocresol poisoning. *Lancet*, **i**, 794–795.

Bidstrup, P. L., Bonnell, J. A. and Beckett, A. G. (1953). Paralysis following poisoning by a new organic phosphorus insecticide (Mipafox). *Brit. Med. J.*, **2**, 1068–1072.

Bignami, G., Rosic, N., Michalek, H., Milosevic, M. and Gatti, G. L. (1975). 'Behavioral Toxicity of anticholinesterase agents' in *Behavioral Toxicology*. Editors: B. Weiss and V. G. Laties. Plenum Press—N.Y. and London.

Bishop, Y., Fujii, K., Arnold, E. and Epstein, S. S. (1971). Censored distribution techniques in analysis of toxicological data. *Experientia*, **27**, 1056–1059.

Biskind, M. S. and Mobbs, R. F. (1972). Psychiatric manifestations from insecticide exposure. *J. Amer. Med. Assoc.*, **220**, 1248.

Blackmore, D. K. (1963). The toxicity of some chlorinated hydrocarbon insecticides to British wild foxes (*Vulpes vulpes*). *J. Comp. Path. Therap.*, **73**, 391–409.

124

Blank, I. H. and Scheuplein, R. J. (1964). 'The Epidermal Barrier' in *Progress in the Biological Sciences in Relation to Dermatology*. Vol. 2. Editors: Rook and Champion. Cambridge University Press—Cambridge.

Blank, I. H., Griesemer, R. D. and Gould, E. (1957). The penetration of an anticholinesterase agent (Sarin) into skin. *J. Invest. Dermatol.*, **29**, 299–309.

Bliss, C. I. (1935a). The comparison of dosage–mortality data. *Ann. Appl. Biol.*, **22**, 306–333.

Bliss, C. I. (1935b). The calculation of the dosage–mortality curve. *Ann. Appl. Biol.*, **22**, 134–167.

Bliss, C. I. (1938). The determination of the dosage–mortality curve from small numbers. *Quart. J. Pharm. Pharmacol.*, **11**, 192–216.

Bliss, C. I. (1940). The relation between exposure time, concentration and toxicity in experiments on insecticides. *Ann. Entomol. Soc. Am.*, **33**, 721–766.

Bliss, C. I. (1957). Some principles of bioassay. *American Scientist*, **45**, 449–466.

Bliss, C. I. (1964). 'Insecticide assays' in *Statistics and Mathematics in Biology*. Editors: O. Kempthorne, T. A. Bancroft, J. W. Gowen and J. L. Lish. Hafner Publishing Co.—N.Y.

Bojanowska, A. and Brzezicka-Bak, M. (1967). Acute and subacute toxicity of dieldrin, administered percutaneously (in Polish). *Rocz, Panstw. Zakl. Hig.*, **18**, 161–169. (*C.A.* 1967, **67**, No. 72787).

Borgmann, U. (1974). A theoretical description of biological rates. *J. theor. Biol.*, **45**, 171–182.

Borison, H. L. and Wang, S. C. (1953). Physiology and pharmacology of vomiting. *Pharmacol. Revs.*, **5**, 193–230.

Borison, H. L., Snow, S. R., Longnecheker, D. S. and Smith, R. P. (1975). 3-chloro-p-toluidine: Effects of lethal doses in rats and cats. *Tox. Appl. Pharmacol.*, **31**, 403–412.

Borowitz, J. L., Moore, P. F., Yim, G. K. W. and Miya, T. S. (1971). Mechanism of enhanced drug effects produced by dilution of the oral dose. *Tox. Appl. Pharmacol.*, **19**, 164–168.

Borredon, I. J. (1970). L'Aeronautique agricole et sa pathologie. *Presse Therm. Climat.*, **108**, 239–243.

Bosquet, W. F., Rupe, B. D. and Miya, T. S. (1965). Endocrine modification of drug responses in the rat. *J. Pharmac. exptl. Ther.*, **147**, 376–379.

Box, G. E. P. (1954). The exploration and exploitation of response surfaces: Some general considerations and examples. *Biometrics*, **10**, 16–60.

Boyd, E. M. (1972). *Predictive Toxicometrics*. Scientechnica Publishers Ltd—Bristol.

Boyd, E. M., Dobos, I. and Krijnen, C. J. (1970). Endosulfan toxicity and dietary protein. *Arch. Environ. Hlth.*, **21**, 15–19.

Braun, H. A. and Lusky, L. M. (1960). The effect of acclimatization to cold on the action of drugs in the rat. *Tox. Appl. Pharmacol.*, **2**, 458–463.

Bray, H. G. and White, K. (1966). *Kinetics and Thermodynamics in Biochemistry*. Churchill—London.

Brittain, R. T. and Spencer, P. J. S. (1965). Use of time–response relationships in assessing pharmacological activity. *J. Pharmacol.*, **17**, 389–391.

Brodeur, J. and Dubois, K. P. (1963). Comparison of acute toxicity of anticholinesterase insecticides to weanling and adult male rats. *Proc. Soc. Exptl Biol. Med.*, **114**, 509–511.

Brodeur, J. and Dubois, K. P. (1964). Studies on the mechanism of acquired tolerance by rats to *o,o*-diethyl-*S*-2-(ethylthio)ethyl phosphorodithioate (Di-Syston). *Arch. int. Pharmacodyn.*, **149**, 560–570.

Brodeur, J. and Dubois, K. P. (1967). Studies on factors influencing the acute toxicity of malathion and malaoxon in rats. *Can. J. Physiol. Pharmacol.*, **45**, 621–631.

Brodie, B. B. and Hogben, C. A. M. (1957). Some physico-chemical factors in drug action. *J. Pharm. Pharmacol.*, **9**, 345–380.

Brody, S. (1964). *Bioenergetics and Growth*. Hafner Publishing Inc.—N.Y.

Brody, T. M. (1955). The uncoupling of oxidative phosphorylation as a mechanism of drug action. *Pharmacol. Rev.*, **7**, 335–363.

Bross, I. (1950). Estimates of the LD_{50}: A critique. *Biometrics*, **6**, 413–423.

Bross, I. D. J. (1958). How to use RIDIT analysis. *Biometrics*, **14**, 18–38.

Brown, A. M. (1961). Sleeping time response of time—random bred, inbred and F_1-hybrids to pentobarbitone sodium. *J. Pharm. Pharmacol.*, **13**, 679–687.

Brown, A. M. (1964). 'Strain and sex differences in response to drugs' in *Evaluation of Drug Activities: Pharmacometrics*. Editors: D. R. Laurence and A. L. Bacharach. Academic Press—London and N.Y.

125

Brown, A. M. (1965). Pharmacogenetics of the mouse. *Lab. Animal Care*, **15**, 111–118.

Brown, B. W. (1966). Planning a quantal assay of potency. *Biometrics*, **22**, 322–329.

Brown, E. A. B. (1974). The localization, metabolism and effects of drugs and toxicants in lung. *Drug. Metab. Rev.*, **3**, 33–87.

Brown, N. C. (1970). *A Review of the Toxicology of Piperonyl Butoxide*. Report A28/52 for Cooper Technical Bureau and The Wellcome Foundation Ltd.

Brown, V. K. H. (1964). The epidermal barrier in toxicology. *Proceedings 2nd International Dermatology Symposium* (Brno—CSSR).

Brown, V. K. H. (1965). Some aspects of percutaneous toxicity testing. *Proceedings 17th International Crop Protection Symposium* (Ghent—Belgium).

Brown, V. K. H. (1966). Laboratory animals for dermatological research. *J. Inst. Animal Tech.*, **17**, 122–126.

Brown, V. K. H. (1968). Solubility and solvent effects as rate determining factors in the acute percutaneous toxicities of pesticides. Society of Chemical Industry, *Monograph No. 29*.

Brown, V. K. H. (1974). Predictive avian toxicity tests with agricultural chemicals. *Proceedings 16th Meeting European Society for the Study of Drug Toxicity* (Carlsbad—CSSR).

Brown, V. K. H. and Box, V. L. (1971). Influence of some solvents on the vascularity of skin in relation to effects on systemic intoxication by solutes. *Proceedings 13th Meeting European Society for the Study of Drug Toxicity* (Berlin—Germany).

Brown, V. K. H. and Muir, C. M. C. (1971). Some factors affecting the acute toxicity of pesticides to mammals when absorbed through skin and eyes. *Int. Pest Control*, **13**, 16–21.

Brown, V. K. H., Robinson, J. and Stevenson, D. E. (1963). A note on the toxicity and solvent properties of dimethyl sulphoxide. *J. Pharm. Pharmacol.*, **15**, 688–692.

Brown, V. K. H., Hunter, C. G. and Richardson, A. (1964). A blood test diagnostic of exposure to aldrin and dieldrin. *Br. J. industr. Med.*, **21**, 283–286.

Brown, V. K. H., Robinson, J. and Richardson, A. (1967a). Preliminary studies on the acute and subacute toxicities of a photoisomerisation product of HEOD. *Fd. Cosmet. Toxicol.*, **5**, 771–779.

Brown, V. K. H., Stevenson, D. E. and Walker, A. I. T. (1967b). Toxicological studies with the molluscicide *N*-tritylmorpholine. *Bull. Wld Hlth Org.*, **37**, 73–77.

Brownleee, K. A., Hodges, J. L. and Rosenblatt, M. (1953). The up-and-down method with small samples. *J. Amer. Statist. Ass.*, **48**, 262–277.

Brus, R. and Herman, Z. S. (1971). Acute toxicities of adrenaline, noradrenaline and acetylcholine in adults and in neo-natal mice. *Dissert. Pharm. Pharmacol.*, **23**, 435–437.

Buck, W. B. (1975). Toxic materials and neurologic disease in cattle. *J. Amer. Vet. Med. Ass.*, **166**, 222–226.

Buerger, A. A. (1967). A theory of integumental penetration. *J. theor. Biol.*, **14**, 66–73.

Buettner, K. J. (1963). The role of the skin barrier layers. *Proc. Sci. Sect. T.G.A.* (No. 40), 8–11.

Buffa, P., Guarriero-Bobyleva, V. and Costa-Tiozzo, R. (1973). Metabolic effect of fluoroacetate poisoning in animals. *Fluoride*, **6**, 224–247.

Bullivant, C. M. (1966). Accidental poisoning by paraquat. *Brit. Med. J.*, **1**, 1272–1273.

Bunning, E. (1967). *The Physiological Clock*, Longmans—London.

Bunyan, P. J. and Taylor, A. (1966). Esterase inhibition in pheasants poisoned by *o,o*-diethyl-*S*-(ethyl-thiomethyl)-phosphorodithioate (Thimet). *J. Agr. Food Chem.*, **14**, 132–137.

Bunyan, P. J., Jennings, D. M. and Jones, F. J. S. (1971). Organophosphorus poisoning: A comparative study of the toxicity of chlorfenvinphos to the pigeon, the pheasant and the Japanese quail. *Pesticide Sci.*, **2**, 148–151.

Burger, Jr, E. J. (1976). *Protecting the Nation's Health*. Lexington Books—Massachussetts and Toronto.

Burton, J. A., Gardiner, T. H. and Schanker, L. S. (1974). Absorption of herbicides from the rat lung. *Arch. Environ. Hlth.*, **29**, 31–33.

Bustad, L. K. and Burns, M. P. (1966). (Editors) Swine in biomedical research. *Proc. Symp. sponsored by U.S. Atomic Energy Commission and The Battelle Memorial Institute, Washington D.C.* July, 1965.

Butler, P. A. (1965). Effects of herbicides on estuarine fauna. *Proc. Southern Weed Conf.*, **18**, 576–580.

Calderbank, A. (1968). The bipyridylium herbicides. *Advances in Pest Control Research*, **8**, 127–235.

126

Caldwell, J., Williams, R. T., Bassir, O. and French, M. R. (1978). Drug metabolism in 'exotic' animals. *Europ. J. Drug Metab. Pharmacok.*, **3**, 61–66.
Camargo, L. A. A., Saad, W. A. and Larini, L. (1970). Acute toxicity of the fenitrothion. *Arg. Inst. Biol. S. Paulo*, **37**, 219–222.
Cann, H. M. (1963). A symposium on pesticides: Pesticide poisoning accidents among young children. *Am. J. Pub. Health*, **53**, 1418–1426.
Carbone, M. G., Sherman, L., Barrow, G. T., McPeak, J., Hook, M. R. and Pickard, R. K. (1976). Organophosphate poisoning in dogs and cats (A panel report). *Mod. Vet. Pract.*, **57**, 638–642.
Carlsson, A. and Serin, F. (1950a). Time of day as a factor influencing the toxicity of nikethamide. *Acta Pharmacol.*, **6**, 181–186.
Carlsson, A. and Serin, F. (1950b). The toxicity of nikethamide at different times of the day. *Acta Pharmacol.*, 187–193.
Carlton, W. W. (1967). Iproniazid-induced encephalopathy in ducklings and chicks. *Exptl. Mol. Path.*, **7**, 133–144.
Carlton, W. W. and Kreutzberg, G. (1966). Isonicotinic acid hydrazide induced spongy degeneration of the white matter in the brains of Pekin ducks. *Amer. J. Path.*, **48**, 91–105.
Carr, Jr, E. A. (1967). Extrapolation of pharmacologic data: Lower animals to man. *Fed. Proc.*, **26**, 1089–1096.
Cartter, M. A. (1961). The cutaneous exposure to PHOSDRIN: Studies on absorption and treatment of intoxication. *Proceedings 13th International Crop Protection Symposium* (Ghent—Belgium).
Casida, J. E. and Baron, R. L. (1976). 'Recognition and overview of the organophosphorus delayed neurotoxicity problem'. *Proceedings of a Symposium on Neurotoxicity held in Washington, D.C.* (Office of Research and Development, Health Effects Research Lab., N.C., U.S.A.).
Casida, J. E. and Sanderson, D. M. (1963). Reaction of certain phosphorothionate insecticides with alcohols and potentiation by breakdown products. *J. Agr. Food Chem.*, **11**, 91–96.
Casida, J. E., Baron, K. L., Eto, M. and Engel, J. L. (1963). Potentiation of neurotoxicity induced by certain organophosphates. *Biochem. Pharmacol.*, **12**, 73–83.
Cavagna, G. and Vigliani, E. C. (1970). Hygienic and safety problems in the use of VAPONA insecticide in domestic situations. *Med. Lavoro*, **61**, 409–423.
Cavagna, G., Locati, G. and Vigliani, E. C. (1969). Clinical effects of exposure to DDVP (VAPONA) insecticide in hospital wards. *Arch. Environ. Health*, **19**, 112–123.
Cavagna, G., Locati, G. and Vigliani, E. C. (1970). Exposure of new-born babies to VAPONA insecticide. *Europ. J. Toxicol.*, **3**, 49–57.
Cavelli, R. D. and Fletcher, K. (1977). 'An effective treatment for paraquat poisoning' in *Biochemical Mechanisms of Paraquat Poisoning*. Editor: A. P. Autor. Academic Press—N.Y. and London.
Chadwick, R. W. and Freal, J. J. (1972). Comparative acceleration of lindane metabolism to chlorophenols by pretreatment of rats with lindane or DDT and lindane. *Fd Cosmet. Toxicol.*, **10**, 789–795.
Chance, M. R. A. (1947). Factors influencing the toxicity of sympathomimetic amines to solitary mice. *J. Pharmacol. exptl. Ther.*, **89**, 289–296.
Chance, M. R. A. and Mackintosh, J. H. (1962). The effects of caging. *Coll. Pap. Lab. Anim. Bur.*, **11**, 59–64.
Chang, M. C., Hunt, D. M. and Turbyfill, C. (1964). High resistance of Mongolian gerbils to irradiation. *Nature*, **203**, 536–537.
Chapman, S. K. and Leibman, K. C. (1971). The effect of chlordane, DDT and 3-methylcholanthrene upon the metabolism and toxicity of parathion. *Tox. Appl. Pharmacol.*, **18**, 977–987.
Choi, S. C. (1971). An investigation of Wetherill's method of estimation for the up-and-down experiment. *Biometrics*, **27**, 961–970.
Christophers, E. and Kligman, A. M. (1964). 'Percutaneous absorption in aged skin' in *Advances in Biology of Skin* Vol. 6. Editor: Montagna. Pergamon Press—Oxford.
Clark, D. G. (1971). Inhibition of the absorption of paraquat from the gastro-intestinal tract by adsorbents. *Brit. J. industr. Med.*, **28**, 186–188.
Clark, D. G. (1973). The toxicological evaluation of aerosols. *Proceedings, 15th Meeting, European Society for the Study of Drug Toxicity* (Zurich—Switzerland).
Clark, D. G., McElligott, T. F. and Hurst, E. W. (1966). The toxicity of paraquat. *Br. J. industr. Med.*, **23**, 126–132.

Clark, D. G. and Hurst, E. W. (1970). The toxicity of diquat. *Br. J. industr. Med.*, **27**, 51–55.

Clark, G. (1971). Organophosphate insecticides and behaviour: A review. *Aerospace Med.*, **42**, 735–740.

Clarke, E. G. C. and Clarke, M. L. (1975). *Veterinary Toxicology*. Bailliere, Tindall and Cassell—London.

Clarke, R. D. (1950). A bio-actuarial approach to forecasting rates of mortality. *Proc. Centen. Assembl. Inst. Actu.*, **2**, 12–27.

Clausing, P. and Bieleke, R. (1979). Methodic aspects of the investigation of coergistic effects in acute oral toxicity. 21st Congress of the European Society of Toxicology (Dresden, DDR). Proceedings to be published.

Clayton, J. W. (1967). Fluorocarbon toxicity: Past, present and future. *J. Soc. Cosmet. Chem.*, **18**, 333–350.

Clendenning, W. E. and Stoughton, R. R. (1962). Importance of the aqueous/lipid partition coefficient for percutaneous absorption of weak electrolytes. *J. Invest. Derm.*, **39**, 47–49.

Coble, Y. P., Hildebrandt, J., Davis, F., Raasch, F. and Curley, A. (1967). Acute endrin poisoning. *J. Amer. Med. Assoc.*, **202**, 489–493.

Cochran, W. G. and Davis, M. (1964). 'Stochastic approximation to the median effective dose in bioassay' in *Stochastic Models in Medicine and Biology*. Editor: J. Gurland. Univ. of Wisconsin Press.

Cohen, G. M. and Mannering, G. J. (1974). Sex-dependent differences in drug metabolism in the rat III. Temporal changes in Type 1 binding and NADPH-cytochrome P-450 reductase during sexual maturation. *Drug. Metab. Dis.*, **2**, 285–292.

Coleman-Cooke, J. (1965). *The Harvest that Kills*. Odhams Books Ltd.—London.

Collins, R. P. (1965). Methyl bromide poisoning: A bizarre neurological disorder. *Calif. Med.*, **103**, 112–115.

Comer, S. W., Staiff, D. C., Armstrong, J. F. and Wolfe, H. R. (1975). Exposure of workers to carbaryl. *Bull. Environ. Contam. Toxicol.*, **13**, 385–391.

Conney, A. H., Welch, R. M., Kuntzman, R. and Burns, J. J. (1967). Effects of pesticides on drug and steroid metabolism. *Clin. Pharmacol. Therap.*, **8**, 2–10.

Conney, A. H., Chang, R., Levin, W. M., Garbut, A., Munro-Faure, A. D., Peck, A. W. and Bye, A. (1972). Effects of piperonyl butoxide on drug metabolism in rodents and man. *Arch. Environ. Health*, **24**, 97–106.

Conyers, R. A. J. and Goldsmith, L. E. (1971). A case of organophosphorus-induced psychosis. *Med. J. Aust.*, **58**, 27–29.

Cook, J. W., Blake, J. R. and Williams, M. W. (1957). The enzymatic hydrolysis of malathion and its inhibition by EPON and other organic phosphorus compounds. *J. Assoc. Off. Agr. Chem.*, **40**, 664–665.

Cook, J. W., Blake, J. R., Yip, G. and Williams, M. W. (1958). Malathionase. I. Activity and inhibition. *J. Assoc. Off. Agr. Chem.*, **41**, 399–411.

Cooke, A. S. (1972). The effects of DDT, dieldrin and 2,4-D on amphibian spawn and tadpoles. *Environ. Pollut.*, **3**, 51–68.

Cooke, M. A. (1965). The problem of skin cleansing. *Trans. St. John's Hosp. derm. Soc. (Lond.)*, **51**, 7–28.

Cooper, E. R. (1976). Pharmacokinetics of skin penetration. *J. Pharm. Sci.*, **65**, 1396–1397.

Cope, O. B. (1961). Standards for reporting fish toxicity tests. *Progressive Fish Culturist*, **23**, 187–189.

Cope, O. B. (1964) Agricultural chemicals and freshwater ecological systems. *Proc. Res. Conf. Pestic.*, Davis, Calif.

Cope, O. B. (1965). Some responses of freshwater fish to herbicides. *Proc. Southern Weed Conf.*, **18**, 439–445.

Copplestone, J. F., Fakhri, Z. I., Miles, J. W., Mitchell, C. A., Osman, Y. and Wolfe, H. R. (1976). Exposure to pesticides in agriculture: A survey of spraymen using dimethoate in the Sudan. *Bull. Wld Hlth Org.*, **54**, 217–223.

Cornfield, J. (1964). 'Measurement and comparison of toxicities: The quantal response' in *Statistics and Mathematics in Biology*. Editors: O. Kempthorne, T. A. Bancroft, J. W. Gowen and J. L. Lush. Hofner Publishing Co.—N.Y.

Cornwell, P. B. (1969). Alphakill—a new rodenticide for mouse control. *Pharm. J.*, **202**, 74–75.

Cornwell, P. B. and Bull, J. O. (1967). Alphakill—a new rodenticide for mouse control. *Pest Control*, **35**, 31–32.

Crabtree, H. C. and Rose, M. S. (1978). Effect of diquat dichloride on gastric emptying and

128

fluid accumulation in the rat stomach. 17th Annual Meeting, Society of Toxicology. (San Francisco, March, 1978)—Abstract only.

Crabtree, H. C., Lock, E. A. and Rose, M. S. (1977). The effect of diquat on the gastrointestinal tract of rats. *Proc. 16th Annual Meeting of the Society of Toxicology.* (Toronto—Canada). (Abstract only).

Craig, F. N., Cummings, E. G. and Sim, V. M. (1977). Environmental temperature and the percutaneous absorption of a cholinesterase inhibitor VX. *J. Invest. Derm.*, **68**, 357–361.

Craig, P. N. (1973). 'Comparison of Hansch and Free-Wilson approaches to structure activity correlations' in *Biological Correlations—The Hansch Approach*. Editor: R. F. Gould. *Advances in Chemistry*, **114**, 115–129.

Craver, B. N., Barrett, W. A. and Earl, A. E. (1950). Some requisites to making LD_{50}'s from different laboratories comparable. *Arch. industr. Hyg. Occup. Med.*, **2**, 280–283.

Crawford, D. L., Sinnhuber, R. O., Stout, F. M., Oldfield, J. E. and Kaufmes, J. K. (1965). Acute toxicity of malonaldehyde. *Tox. Appl. Pharmacol.*, **7**, 826–832.

Cremer, J. E. and Bligh, J. (1969). Body temperature and responses to drugs. *Brit. Med. Bull.*, **23**, 299–306.

Cronin, E. and Stoughton, R. B. (1962). Percutaneous absorption: Regional variations and the effect of hydration and epidermal stripping. *Br. J. Derm.*, **74**, 265–272.

Crook, J. H. and Ward, P. (1968). 'The Quelea problem in Africa' in *The Problems of Birds as Pests*. Editors: R. K. Murton and E. N. Wright. Academic Press—London and N.Y.

Crossland, J. and Shea, K. P. (1973). The hazards of impurities. *Environment*, **15**, 35–38.

Crossland, N. O. and Elgar, K. E. (1974). Evaluation of the side-effects of the herbicide WL 63611 in aquatic ecosystems. *Proc. 4th Int. Symp. on Aquatic Weeds (Vienna)*.

Crounse, R. G. (1965). Keratin and the barrier. *Arch. Environ. Health*, **11**, 522–528.

Cueto, Jr., C. and Biros, F. J. (1967). Chlorinated insecticides and related materials in human urine. *Tox. Appl. Pharmacol.*, **10**, 261–269.

Cummings, E. G. (1969). Temperature and concentration effects on penetration of N-octylamine through human skin *in situ. J. Invest. Derm.*, **53**, 64–70.

Curley, A., Sedlak, V. A., Girling, E. F., Hawk, R. E., Barthel, W. F., Pierce, P. E. and Likosky, W. H. (1971). Organic mercury identified as the cause of poisoning in humans and hogs. *Science*, **172**, 65–67.

Damluji, S. F. and Tikriti, S. (1972). Mercury poisoning from wheat. *Br. Med. J.*, **i**, 804 only.

Daniel, J. W. and Gage, J. C. (1966). Absorption and excretion of diquat and paraquat in rats. *Brit. J. industr. Med.*, **23**, 133–136.

Daum, R. J. and Killcreas, W. (1966). Two computer programs for probit analysis. *Bull. Entomol. Soc. Amer.*, **12**, 365–369.

Dauterman, W. C. (1971). Biological and non-biological modifications of organophosphorus compounds. *Bull. Wld Hlth Org.*, **44**, 133–150.

Davies, G. M. and Lewis, I. (1956). Outbreak of food poisoning from bread made of chemically contaminated flour. *Br. Med. J.*, **ii**, 393–398.

Davies, J. E. (1972). Effects of different types of exposure of different kinds of pesticides on man as determined through laboratory testing. *Proc. Nat. Conf. on Protective Clothing and Safety Equipment for Pesticide Workers (Federal Working Group on Pest. Management)*. Rockville, Md., U.S.A

Davies, J. E. and Edmundson, W. F. (1972). Editors *Epidemiology of DDT*. Futura Publishing Co. Inc.—N.Y.

Davies, J. E., Barquet, A., Freed, V. H., Haque, R., Morgade, C., Sonnelborn, R. E. and Vaclaver, C. (1975). Human pesticide poisoning by a fat-soluble organophosphate insecticide. *Arch. Environ. Hlth.*, **30**, 608–613.

Davies, R. G. (1971). *Computer Programming in Quantitative Biology*. Academic Press—London and N.Y.

Davis, R. A. (1970). 'Control of rats and mice' in *U.K. Ministry of Agriculture, Fisheries and Food Bulletin No. 181*. HMSO—London.

Davis, R. J. and Davies, B. H. (1970). The biochemistry of warfarin resistance in the rat. *Biochem. J.*, **118**, 44P–45P.

Davis, W. M. (1962). Day–night periodicity in pentobarbital response of mice and the influence of socio-psychological conditions. *Experientia*, **18**, 235–237.

Dean, B. J. and Thorpe, E. (1972). Studies with dichlorvos vapours in dominant lethal mutations tests on mice. *Arch. Toxicol.*, **30**, 51–60.

De Beer, E. J. (1945). The calculation of biological assay results by graphic methods. The all-or-none type of response. *J. Pharmacol. exptl. Therap.*, **85**, 1–13.

Dedrick, R. L. (1974). Animal scale-up. *J. Pharmacokin. Biopharm.*, **1**, 435–461.

Deichman, W. B. and Mergard, E. G. (1948). Evaluation of methods employed to express the degree of toxicity of a compound. *J. industr. Hyg. Toxicol.*, **30**, 373–378.

De Jongh, S. E. (1961). 'Isoboles' in *Quantitative Methods in Pharmacology*. Editor: H. de Jonge. North-Holland Publishing Co.—Amsterdam.

De Lopez, O. H., Smith, F. A. and Hodge, H. C. (1976). Plasma fluoride concentrations in rats acutely poisoned with sodium fluoride. *Tox. Appl. Pharmacol.*, **37**, 75–83.

De Palma, A. E., Kwalick, D. S. and Zukerberg, N. (1970). Pesticide poisoning in children. *J. Amer. Med. Assoc.*, **211**, 1979–1981.

Derban, L. K. A. (1974). Outbreak of food poisoning due to alkyl-mercury fungicide on Southern Ghana State Farm. *Arch. Environ. Health*, **28**, 49–52.

Derome, J. R. (1977). Biological similarity and group theory. *J. theor. Biol.*, **65**, 369–378.

Desi, I., Dura, G., Szlobodnyik, J. and Csuka, I. (1977). Testing of pesticide toxicity in tissue culture. *J. Tox. environ. Hlth.*, **2**, 1053–1066.

De Witt, J. B. (1966). Methodology for determining toxicity of pesticides to wild vertebrates. *J. Appl. Ecol.*, **3** (Supp.), 275–278.

Dews, P. B. and Berkson, J. (1964). 'On the error of bio-assay with quantal response' in *Statistics and Mathematics in Biology*. Editors: O. Kempthorne, T. A. Bencroft, J. W. Gowen and J. L. Lush. Hafner Publishing Co.—N.Y.

Dieke, S. H. and Richter, C. P. (1945). Acute toxicity of thiourea to rats in relation to age, diet, strain and species variation. *J. Pharmac. exptl. Ther.*, **83**, 195–202.

Dieterich, R. A. (1975). The collared lemming (*Dicrostonyx stevensoni* Nelson) in biomedical research. *Lab. Anim. Sci.*, **25**, 48–54.

Dikshith, T. S. S., Datta, K. K. and Chandra, P. (1974). Interaction of lindane and diazinon on the skin of rats. *Exp. Pathol.*, **9**, 219–224.

Dinman, B. D. (1972). 'Non-concept' of 'No-threshold': Chemicals in the environment. *Science*, **175**, 495–497.

Dixon, R. L. (1976). Problems in extrapolating toxicity data for laboratory animals to men. *Environ. Hlth Perspect.*, **13**, 43–50.

Dixon, R. L., Adamson, R. H. and Rall, D. P. (1966). Toxicity and pharmacology of an unusual solvent: tetramethylurea. *Arch. int. Pharmacodyn.*, **160**, 333–341.

Dixon, W. J. (1965). The up and down method for small samples. *J. Amer. statist. Ass.*, **60**, 967–978.

Dollery, C. T., Davies, D. S. and Connolly, M. E. (1971). Differences in the metabolism of drugs depending on their route of administration. *Ann. N.Y. Acad. Sci.*, **179**, 108–114.

Doluisio, J. T., Billups, N. F., Dittert, L. W., Sugita, F. T. and Swintosky, J. V. (1969a). Drug absorption 1. An *in situ* rat gut technique yielding realistic absorption rates. *J. Pharm. Sci.*, **58**, 1196–1200.

Doluisio, J. T., Tan, G. H., Billups, N. F. and Diamond, L. (1969b). Drug absorption II: Effect of fasting on intestinal drug absorption. *J. Pharm. Sci.*, **58**, 1200–1204.

Done, A. K. (1964). Developmental pharmacology. *Clin. Pharmacol. Therap.*, **5**, 432–479.

Done, A. K. and Peart, A. J. (1971). Acute toxicities of arsenical herbicides. *Clin. Tox.*, **4**, 343–355.

Donninger, C. (1971). Species specificity of phosphate triester anticholinesterases. *Bull. Wld Hlth Org.*, **44**, 265–268.

Doull, J. (1972). 'The effect of physical environmental factors on drug response' in *Essays in Toxicology*, Vol. 3. Editor: W. J. Hayes, Jr. Academic Press—N.Y. and London.

Dowden, B. F. and Bennett, H. J. (1965). Toxicity of selected chemicals to certain animals. *J. Water Pollut. Control Fed.*, **37**, 1308–1316.

Draize, J. H. (1959). 'Dermal toxicity' in *Appraisal of the Safety of Chemicals in Foods, Drugs and Cosmetics*. Editors: Staff of Division of Pharmacology of Food and Drug Administration, U.S. Dept. of Health, Education and Welfare. (Association of Food and Drug Officials of the United States.)

Draize, J. H., Nelson, A. A. and Calvery, H. O. (1944). The percutaneous absorption of DDT in laboratory animals. *J. Pharm. exptl Ther.*, **82**, 159–166.

Drenth, H. J., Ensberg, I. F. G., Roberts, D. V. and Wilson, A. (1972). Neuromuscular function in agricultural workers using pesticides. *Arch. Environ. Health*, **25**, 395–398.

Drew, R. T. and Laskin, S. (1973). 'Environmental inhalation chambers' in *Methods of Animal Experimentation* Vol. 4. Editor: W. I. Gray. Academic Press—N.Y. and London.

130

DuBois, K. P. (1958). Potentiation of the toxicity of insecticidal organic phosphates. *Arch. Industr. Health*, **18**, 488–496.

DuBois, K. P. (1961). Potentiation of the toxicity of organophosphorus compounds. *Advances in Pest Control Research*, **4**, 117–151.

DuBois, K. P. (1963). 'Toxicological evaluation of anticholinesterase agents' in *Handbuck der Experimentellen Pharmacologie* Vol. 15. Editor: G. B. Koelle. Springer-Verlag—Berlin.

DuBois, K. P. (1971). The toxicity of organophosphorus compounds to mammals. *Bull. Wld Hlth Org.*, **44**, 233–240.

DuBois, K. P., Doull, J., Salerno, P. R. and Coon, J. M. (1949). Studies on the toxicity and mechanism of action of *p*-nitrophenyl diethyl thionophosphate (parathion). *J. Pharmacol. exptl. Ther.*, **95**, 79–91.

Dudley, A. W. and Thaoar, N. Y. (1972). Fatal human ingestion of 2,4-D, a common herbicide. *Arch. Path.*, **94**, 270–275.

Duffy, B. S. and O'Sullivan, D. J. (1968). Paraquat poisoning. *J. Irish Med. Assoc.*, **61**, 97–98.

Dunnett, C. W. (1968). 'Biostatistics in pharmacological testing' in *Selected Pharmacological Testing Methods*. Editor: A. Burger. Edward Arnold (Publishers) Ltd.—London.

Durham, W. F. and Wolfe, H. R. (1962). Measurement of the exposure of workers to pesticides. *Bull. Wld Hlth Org.*, **26**, 75–91.

Durham, W. F., Wolfe, H. R. and Quinby, G. E. (1965). Organophosphorus insecticides and mental alertness. *Arch. Environ. Hlth.*, **10**, 55–66.

Durham, W. F., Wolfe, H. R. and Elliott, J. W. (1972). Absorption and excretion of parathion by spraymen. *Arch. Environ. Hlth*, **24**, 381–387.

Eben, A. and Pilz, W. (1967). Abhangigbeit der Acetylcholinesterase-acktivatät in Plasma and Erythrocyten von alter und geschlecht der Ratte. *Arch. Toxicol.*, **23**, 27–34.

Edery, H. and Schatzberg-Porath, G. (1960). Studies on the effect of organophosphorus insecticides on amphibians. *Arch. int. Pharmacodyn.*, **124**, 212–224.

Editorial (1964). The fluoroacetamide episode. *Fd. Cosmet. Toxicol.*, **2**, 381–382.

Ehrlich, P. R. and Ehrlich, A. H. (1970). *Population, Resources, Environment—Issues in Human Ecology*. W. H. Freeman & Co.—San Francisco.

Eichhorn, B. H. (1972). Sequential search of an optimal dosage II. Technical Report No. 5, Dept. of Mathematics and Statistics, Case Western University, Cleveland, Ohio, U.S.A.

Eichhorn, B. H. and Zacks, S. (1972). Sequential search of an optimal dosage: I. Some preliminary results and suggested areas for further research. Technical Report No. 3, Dept. of Mathematics and Statistics, Case Western University, Cleveland, Ohio, U.S.A.

Eickholt, T. H. and White, W. F. (1960). The toxicity and absorption enhancing ability of surfactants. *Drug. Stand.*, **28**, 154–161.

Elias, P. M. (1975). Permeability barriers and pathways in mammalian epidermis. Paper presented to joint meeting of the Society of Investigative Dermatology Inc. and the European Society for Dermatological Research—Amsterdam, June, 1975. (Abstract only published).

Elias, P. M., Goerke, J. and Friend, D. S. (1977). Mammalian epidermal layer lipids composition and influence on structure. *J. Invest. Derm.*, **69**, 535–546.

Elliott, J. W., Walker, K. C., Penick, A. E. and Durham, W. F. (1960). Insecticide exposure: A sensitive procedure for urinary *p*-nitrophenol determination as a measure of exposure to parathion. *J. Agric. Food Chem.*, **8**, 111–113.

El Masry, S. E. D. and Mannering, G. J. (1974). Sex-dependent differences in drug metabolism in the rat: II. Quantitative changes produced by castration and the administration of steroid hormone and phenobarbital. *Drug. Metab. Disp.*, **2**, 279–284.

El Masry, S. E. D., Cohen, G. M. and Mannering, G. J. (1974). Sex dependent differences in drug metabolism in the rat: I. Temporal changes in the microsomal drug-metabolizing system of the liver during sexual maturation. *Drug. Metab. Disp.*, **2**, 267–278.

Elsea, J. R., Coyd, G. D., Gilbert, D. L., Perkinson, E. and Ward, J. W. (1970). Barbiturate anaesthesia in dogs wearing collars containing dichlorvos. *J.A.V.M.A.*, **157**, 2068.

Emsley, J. (1978). The trouble with thallium. *New Scientist*, **79**, 392–394.

Enslein, K., Knanna, D. and Craig, P. N. (1977). A toxicity prediction system. *Proceedings 16th Annual Meeting of the Society of Toxicology (Toronto—Canada)*. (Abstract only).

Ertel, R. J., Halberg, F. and Ungar, F. (1964). Circadian system phase-dependent toxicity and other effects of methopyrapone (SU 4885) in the mouse. *J. Pharmac. exptl. Ther.*, **146**, 395–399.

Fairshter, R. D. and Wilson, A. F. (1975). Paraquat poisoning—manifestation and therapy. *Amer. J. Med.*, **59**, 751–753.

Farmer, J. (1974). Comparison of probit and logit models for estimation of LD_{01}. *Fed. Proc.*, **33**, 220.

Farnsworth, L. (1977). Observations on the management, breeding and behaviour of European hamsters (*cricetus cricetus*). Paper read at Institute of Animal Technicians' Congress—York, 1977. (To be published).

Faucher, J. A. and Goddard, E. F. (1978). Interaction of keratinous substrates with sodium lauryl sulphate. II. Permeation through stratum corneum. *J. Soc. Cosmet. Chem.*, **29**, 339–352.

Feldmann, R. J. and Maibach, H. I. (1970). Absorption of some organic compounds through the skin in man. *J. Invest. Derm.*, **54**, 399–404.

Feldmann, R. J. and Maibach, H. I. (1974). Percutaneous penetration of some pesticides and herbicides in man. *Tox. Appl. Pharmacol.*, **28**, 126–132.

Felsenstein, W. C., Smith, R. P. and Gosselin, R. E. (1974). Toxicologic studies on the avicide 3-chloro-*p*-toluidine. *Tox. Appl. Pharmacol.*, **28**, 110–125.

Ferguson, H. C. (1962). Dilution of dose and acute oral toxicity. *Tox. Appl. Pharmacol.*, **4**, 759–762.

Ferguson, J. (1939). The use of chemical potentials as indices of toxicity. *Proc. Roy. Soc.*, *(B)*, **127**, 387–404.

Fincher, J. H. (1968). Particle size of drugs and its relationship to absorption and activity. *J. Pharm. Sci.*, **57**, 1825–1835.

Fink, H. and Hund, G. (1965). Probitanalyse mittels programmgesteuerter Rechenanalagen. *Arzneimittellforschung*, **15**, 624–630.

Finney, D. J. (1971). *Probit Analysis*. Cambridge University Press—Cambridge.

Fletcher, K. (1974). 'Paraquat poisoning' in *Forensic Toxicology*. Editor: B. Ballantyne. John Wright and Sons Ltd.—Bristol.

Flynn, E. J., Lynch, M. and Zannoni, V. G. (1972). Species differences and drug metabolism. *Biochem. Pharmacol.*, **21**, 2577–2590.

Fournier, E. (1974). Toxicite humaine des pesticides. *Bull. Soc. Zool. France*, **99**, 39–48.

Franz, T. J. (1975). Percutaneous absorption: on the relevance of *in vitro* data. *J. Invest. Derm.*, **64**, 190–195.

Frawley, J. P. (1965). 'Synergism and Antagonism' in *Research in Pesticides*. Editor: C. O. Chichester. Academic Press—N.Y. and London.

Frawley, J. P., Fuyat, H. N., Hagen, E. C., Blanke, J. R. and Fitzhugh, O. G. (1957). Marked potentiation in mammalian toxicity from simultaneous administration of two anticholinesterase compounds. *J. Pharmacol. exptl Therap.*, **121**, 96–106.

Frazer, A. C. and Sharratt, M. (1969). 'The value and limitations of animal studies in the prediction of effects in man' in *The Use of Animals in Toxicology Studies*. *Proc. UFAW Symp. London*–January 1969.

Fredricksson, T. (1964). Studies on the percutaneous absorption of parathion and paraoxon: (VI) *in vivo* decomposition of paraoxon during epidermal passage. *J. Invest. Derm.*, **42**, 37–40.

Fredriksson, T., Farrior, W. L. and Wittar, R. F. (1961). Studies on the percutaneous absorption of parathion and paraoxon: (I) Hydrolysis and metabolism within the skin. *Acta Dermato-Venereol.*, **41**, 335–343.

Free, Jr., S. M. and Wilson, J. W. (1964). A mathematical contribution to structure-activity studies. *J. Med. Chem.*, **7**, 395–399.

Freed, V. H. and Witt, J. M. (1969). 'Physiochemical principles in formulating pesticides relating to biological activity' in *Pesticidal Formulations Research*. Editor: J. W. van Valkenburg. *Advances in Chemistry Series 86* (American Chemical Society—Washington, D.C.).

Freedland, R. A. (1967). Effect of progressive starvation on rat liver enzyme activities. *J. Nutrition*, **91**, 489–495.

Freedman, A. M. and Himwich, H. E. (1948). Effect of age on lethality of di-isopropyl fluorophosphate. *Am. J. Physiol.*, **153**, 121–126.

Freedman, A. M. and Himwich, H. E. (1949). DFP: Site of injection and variation in response. *Am. J. Physiol.*, **156**, 125–128.

Freireich, E. J., Gehan, E. A., Rall, D. P., Schmidt, L. H. and Skipper, H. E. (1966). Quantitative comparison of toxicity of anticancer agents in mouse, rat, hamster, dog, monkey and man. *Cancer Chemotherapy Reports*, **50**, 219–244.

Friend, M. and Trainer, D. O. (1972). Duck hepatitis virus interactions with DDT and dieldrin in adult mallards. *Bull. Environ. Contam. Tox.*, **7**, 202–205.

132

Fristedt, B. and Sterner, N. (1965). Warfarin intoxication from percutaneous absorption. *Arch. Environ. Hlth*, **11**, 205–208.

Fukami, J., Mitsui, T., Fukunaga, K. and Shishido, T. (1970). 'The selective toxicity of rotenone between mammal, fish and insect' in *Biochemical Toxicology of Insecticides*. Editors: R. D. O'Brien and I. Yamamoto. Academic Press—N.Y. and London.

Funaki, H. (1974). Drug toxicity (LD_{50}) and *dosis medicamentosa* for children in terms of body surface area and body weight (Preliminary Report). *J. Kyoto Pref. Univ. Med.*, **83**, 467–477.

Funckes, A. J., Hayes, Jr., G. R. and Hartwell, W. V. (1963). Urinary excretion of *para*nitrophenol by volunteers following dermal exposure to parathion at different ambient temperatures. *J. Agr. Food Chem.*, **11**, 455–457.

Fytizas, R. (1970). Influence de trois solvants sur la toxicite cutanée aigue et subaigue du DDVP. *Annls. Inst. phytopath. Benaki*, **9**, 245–248.

Gaddum, J. H. (1933). Methods of biological assay depending on a quantal response. *Med. Res. Cncl Spec. Rpt., No. 183*.

Gaines, T. B. (1960). The acute toxicity of pesticides to rats. *Tox. Appl. Pharmacol.*, **2**, 88–99.

Gaines, T. B. (1969). Acute toxicity of pesticides. *Tox. Appl. Pharmacol.*, **14**, 515–534.

Gaines, T. B., Hayes, Jr., W. J. and Linder, R. E. (1966). Liver metabolism of anticholinesterase compounds in live rats: relation to toxicity. *Nature*, **209**, 88–89.

Ganelin, R. S., Cueto, Jr. C. and Mail, G. A. (1964a). Exposure to parathion: Effect on general population and asthmatics. *J. Am. Med. Assoc.*, **188**, 807–810.

Ganelin, R. S., Mail, G. A. and Cueto, C. (1964b). Hazards of equipment contaminated with parathion. *Arch. Environ. Hlth.*, **8**, 826–828.

Gardner, A. L. and Iverson, R. E. (1968). The effect of aerially applied malathion on an urban population. *Arch. Environ. Hlth.*, **16**, 823–826.

Gehlbach, S. H. and Williams, W. A. (1975). Pesticide containers—their contribution to poisoning. *Arch. Environ. Hlth.*, **30**, 49–50.

Gerarde, H. W. (1963). Toxicological studies on hydrocarbons. *Arch. Environ. Hlth.*, **6**, 329–341.

Gerarde, H. W. and Ahlstrom, D. B. (1966). The aspiration hazard and toxicity of a homologous series of alcohols. *Arch. Environ. Hlth.*, **13**, 457–461.

Gerboth, G. and Schwabe, U. (1964). Einfluss von gewebsgespeichertem DDT auf die Wirkung von Pharmaka. *Arch. Exp. Path. u. Pharmak.*, **246**, 469–483.

Gervais, P. (1976). Risque chimique dû aux insecticides: les dosages des cholinesterases et l'hygiène d'usage des organophosphorés. *Arch. Mal. Prof. Med. Trav. Sec. Soc.*, **37**, 320–324.

Gibaldi, M., Boyes, R. N. and Feldman, S. (1971). Influence of first-pass effect on availability of drugs on oral administration. *J. Pharm. Sci.*, **60**, 1338–1340.

Gibson, E. A. (1977). The apparent susceptibility of golden orfe (*Idus idus* var.) to certain agricultural chemicals. *Vet. Rec.*, **100**, 531.

Gingell, R. and Wallcare, L. (1974). Species differences in the acute toxicity and tissue distribution of DDT in mice and hamsters. *Tox. Appl. Pharmacol.*, **28**, 385–394.

Gitelson, S., Davidson, J. T. and Werczberger, A. (1965). Phosphamidon poisoning. *Brit. J. industr. Med.*, **22**, 236–239.

Glow, P. H. and Rose, S. (1965). Effects of reduced acetylcholinesterase levels on extinction of a conditional response. *Nature*, **206**, 475–477.

Gohlke, R. and Grigorowa, R. (1973). Ueber die kombinierte wirkung von phosphororganischen pestiziden und erhoehter umgebungstemperatur in inhalatorischem kurzuersuchen an ralten: II. Histologische, histochemische und morphometrische untersuchungen. *Int. Archiv. Arbeitsmed.*, **31**, 309–327.

Gold, H. J. (1977). *Mathematical Modeling of Biological Systems—an Introductory Guidebook*. John Wiley & Sons—N.Y., London, Sydney and Toronto.

Goldberg, M. E., Johnson, H. E., Knaar, J. B. and Smyth, H. F. (1963). Psychopharmacological effects of reversible cholinesterase inhibition induced by *N*-methyl 3,-isopropyl phenyl carbamate (Compound 10854). *J. Pharmacol. exptl Ther.*, **141**, 244–252.

Goldenthal, E. I. (1971). A compilation of LD_{50} values in newborn and adult animals. *Tox. Appl. Pharmacol.*, **18**, 185–207.

Goldman, H. and Teitel, M. (1958). Malathion poisoning in a 34-month-old child following accidental ingestion. *J. Pediat.*, **52**, 76–81.

133

Goldwater, L. J. (1968). 'Toxicology' in *Dangerous Properties of Industrial Materials*. Editor: N. Irving-Sax. Reinhold Book Corporation—N.Y., Amsterdam, London.

Goodman, L. S. and Gilman, A. (1970). *The Pharmacological Basis of Therapeutics*. Macmillan—New York.

Goodrick, C. L. (1973). The effects of dietary protein upon growth of inbred and hybrid mice. *Growth*, 37, 355–367.

Gordon, J. J., Leadbeater, L. and Maidhent, M. P. (1978). The protection of animals against organophosphate poisoning by pretreatment with a carbamate. *Tox. Appl. Pharmacol.*, 43, 207–216.

Goulding, R. (1969). Current trends in toxicological requirements. *Proc. 5th Br. Insectic. Fungi.Conf.*—Brighton 1969.

Goulding, R., Volans, G. N., Crome, P. and Widdop, B. (1976). Paraquat poisoning. *Br. Med. J.*, 1, 42.

Grant, C. A. (1971). 'Pathology of experimental methymercury intoxication: some problems of exposure and response' in *Mercury, Mercurials and Mercaptans*. Editors: M. W. Miller and T. W. Clarkson. Chas. C. Thomas—Springfield.

Grasso, P. (1971). Some aspects of the role of skin appendages in percutaneous absorption. *J. Soc. Cosmet. Chem.*, 22, 523–534.

Grasso, P. and Lansdown, A. B. G. (1972). Methods of measuring and factors affecting percutaneous absorption. *J. Soc. Cosmet. Chem.*, 23, 481–521.

Gratz, N. G. (1973). A critical review of currently used single dose rodenticides. *Bull. Wld Hlth Org.*, 48, 469–477.

Gray, H. and Addis, T. (1948). Rat colony testing by Zucker's weight–age relation. *Am. J. Physiol.*, 153, 35–40.

Green, C. D. (1968). Strain sensitivity of rats to nitrous oxide. *Anaes. Analg.*, 47, 509–514.

Greene, L. T. (1971). 'Aerosols' in *Handbuck der experimentellen Pharmakologie* Vol. 28 (Pt 1). Editors: B. B. Brodie and J. R. Gillette. Springer-Verlag—Berlin, Heidelberg and N.Y.

Greenwood, D. A. and Ghadiri, M. (1966). Combinations raise insecticide toxicity. *Chem. Eng. News*, 44, (31.1.66), 28 only.

Grice, K., Sattar, H. and Baker, H. (1972). The effect of ambient humidity on transepidermal water loss. *J. Invest. Derm.*, 58, 343–346.

Griffith, J. F. (1964). Interlaboratory variations in the determination of acute oral LD_{50}. *Tox. Appl. Pharmacol.*, 6, 726–730.

Grigorowa, R. and Binnewies, S. (1973). Ueber die kombinierte Wirkung von phosphororganischen pestiziden und erhoehter umgebungstemperatur in inhalatorischen kurzuersuchen an ratten: I. Toxikologische aspekte. *Int. Archiv arbeitsmed.*, 31, 295–307.

Grover, J. (1971). Acute poisoning. *Armed Forces Med. J. (India)*, 27, 358–278.

Guilbault, G. G., Sadar, M. H., Kuan, S. and Casey, D. (1970). Effect of pesticides on liver cholinesterases from rabbit, pigeon, chickens, sheep and pig. *Anal. Chim. Acta*, 51, 83–93.

Guiti, N. and Sadeghi, D. (1969). Acute toxicity of malathion in the mongrel dog. *Tox. Appl. Pharmacol.*, 15, 244–245.

Gurland, J., Lee, I. and Dahm, P. A. (1960). Polychotomous quantal response in biological assay. *Biometrics*, 16, 382–398.

Guthrie, F. E., Monroe, R. J. and Abernathy, C. O. (1971). Response of the laboratory mouse to selection for resistance to insecticides. *Tox. Appl. Pharmacol.*, 18, 92–101.

Guthrie, F. E., Domanski, J. J., Main, A. R., Sanders, D. G. and Monroe, R. R. (1974). Use of mice for initial approximation of re-entry intervals into pesticide treated field. *Arch. Environ. Contam. Toxicol.*, 2, 233–242.

Haber, F. (1924). 'Zur geschichte des gaskriejes' in *Funf Vortrage aus den Jahren 1920–1923*. Julius Springer—Berlin.

Hagan, E. C. (1959). 'Acute toxicity' in *Appraisal of the Safety of Chemicals in Foods, Drugs and Cosmetics*. Association of Food and Drug Officials of the United States.

Halberg, F., Johnson, E. A., Brown, B. W. and Bittner, J. J. (1960). Susceptibility rhythm to *E. coli* endotoxin and bioassay. *Proc. Soc. Exptl. Biol. Med.*, 103, 142–144.

Haley, T. J., Dooley, K. L. and Harmon, J. R. (1973). Acute oral toxicity of *N*-2-fluorenylacetamide (2 FAA) in several strains of mice. *Proc. Soc. Exp. Biol. Med.*, 143, 1117–1119.

Haley, T. J., Farmer, J. H., Dooley, K. L., Harmon, J. R. and Peoples, A. (1974a). Determination of the LD_{01} and extrapolation of the LD_{001} for methylcarbamate pesticides. *Europ. J. Toxicol.*, 7, 152–158.

134

Haley, T. J., Harmon, J. R., Dooley, K. L. and Uhler, R. (1974b). Comparison of the oral LD_{01} of carbaryl and dichlorvos. *Fed. Proc.*, **33**, 230.

Haley, T. J., Farmer, J. H., Harmon, J. R. and Dooley, K. L. (1975a). Estimation of the LD_1 and extrapolation of the $LD_{0.1}$ for five organothiophosphate pesticides. *Europ. J. Toxicol.*, **8**, 229–235.

Haley, T. J., Farmer, J. H., Harmon, J. R. and Dooley, K. L. (1975b). Estimation of the $LD_{0.1}$ for five organophosphate pesticides. *Arch. Toxicol.*, **34**, 103–109.

Hamilton, A. and Hardy, H. L. (1974). 'Pesticides' in *Industrial Toxicology*. Publishing Sciences Group Inc.—Acton, Massachusetts.

Hamilton, G. A., Hunter, K., Ritchie, A. S., Ruthven, A. D., Brown, P. M. and Stanley, P. I. (1976). Poisoning of wild geese by carbophenothion-treated wheat. *Pestic. Sci.*, **7**, 175–183.

Hamza, S. M. (1973). Relationship between depression of blood cholinesterase and paralysis in Egyptian buffaloes by an organophosphorus compound. *Egypt. J. Vet. Sci.*, **10**, 53–63.

Handler, P. (1974). Quoted statement. *Pesticide Chemical News*, **2**, 7.

Hanig, J. P., Yoder, P. D. and Krop, S. (1976). Convulsions in weanling rabbits after a single topical application of 1% lindane. *Tox. Appl. Pharm.*, **38**, 463–469.

Hanninen, O. (1975). Age and exposure factors in drug metabolism. *Acta Pharmacol. Toxicol.*, **36**, Supp. II, 3–20.

Hansch, C. (1970). 'The use of physiochemical parameters and regression analysis in pesticide design' in *Biochemical Toxicology of Pesticides*. Editors: O'Brien and Yamamoto. Academic Press—N.Y. and London.

Harbison, R. D. (1975). Comparative toxicity of some selected pesticides in neonatal and adult rats. *Tox. Appl. Pharmacol.*, **32**, 443–446.

Harbison, R. D. and Koshakji, R. P. (1975). Studies on the mechanism of increased susceptibility of the newborn to parathion toxicity. *Fed. Proc.*, **34**, 245.

Harris, D. R., Paper, C. M. and Stanton, R. (1974). Percutaneous absorption and the surface area of occluded skin. *Brit. J. Derm.*, **91**, 27–32.

Harris, W. S. (1973). Toxic effects of aerosol propellants on the heart. *Arch. Intern. Med.*, **131**, 162–166.

Hart, E. R. (1967). Relationship of effective dose to body weight. Report (unclassified) to U.S. Army Research Office.

Hart, L. G. and Fouts, J. R. (1963). Effects of acute and chronic DDT administration on hepatic microsomal drug metabolism in the rat. *Proc. Soc. Exptl. Biol. Med.*, **114**, 388–392.

Hart, L. G., Shultice, R. W. and Fouts, J. R. (1963). Stimulatory effects of chlordane on hepatic microsomal drug metabolism in the rat. *Tox. Appl. Pharmacol.*, **5**, 371–386.

Hartwell, W. V. and Hayes, Jr. G. R. (1965). Respiratory exposure to organic phosphorus insecticides. *Arch. environ. Hlth.*, **11**, 564–568.

Hartwell, W. V., Hayes, Jr. G. R. and Funckes, A. J. (1964). Respiratory exposure of volunteers to parathion. *Arch. environ. Hlth.*, **8**, 820–825.

Harvey, D. G., Bidstrup, P. L. and Bonnell, J. A. L. (1951). Poisoning by dinitro-orthocresol. *Br. Med. J.*, **2**, 13–18.

Hashimoto, Y., Makita, T., Miyata, H., Noguchi, T. and Ohta, G. (1968). Acute and subchronic toxicity of a new fluorine pesticide, *N*-methyl-*N*-(1-naphthyl fluoroacetamide). *Tox. Appl. Pharmacol.*, **12**, 536–547.

Hatch, T. F. and Gross, P. (1964). *Pulmonary Deposition and retention of Inhaled Aerosols*. Academic Press—N.Y. and London.

Hathway, D. E. (1970). 'Species, strain and sex differences in metabolism' in *Foreign Compound Metabolism in Mammals*. Senior Editor: D. E. Hathway. The Chemical Society—London.

Haus, E. and Halberg, F. (1959). 24-hour rhythm in susceptibility of c-mice to a toxic dose of ethanol. *J. Appl. Physiol.*, **14**, 878–880.

Hayes, Jr., G. R., Funckes, A. J. and Hartwell, M. V. (1964). Dermal exposure of human volunteers to parathion. *Arch. Environ. Hlth.*, **8**, 829–833.

Hayes, Jr. W. J. (1959). The toxicity of dieldrin to man. *Bull. Wld Hlth Org.*, **20**, 891–912.

Hayes, Jr., W. J. (1963). *Clinical Handbook on Economic Poisons*. Environmental Protection Agency, (Pesticide Programs)—Camblee, Georgia, U.S.A.

Hayes, Jr., W. J. (1971). Studies on exposure during the use of anticholinesterase pesticides. *Bull. Wld Hlth Org.*, **44**, 277–288.

Hayes, Jr., W. J. (1974). Distribution of dieldrin following a single oral dose. *Tox. Appl. Pharmacol.*, **28**, 485–492.

Hayes, Jr., W. J. (1975). Mortality from pesticides in 1969. *Tox. Appl. Pharmacol.*, **33**, 145.

Hayes, Jr., W. J. (1977). Mortality in 1973 and 1974 from pesticides. Paper presented at 16th Annual Meeting of Society of Toxicology (Toronto—Canada).

Hayes, Jr., W. J. and Pearce, G. W. (1953). Pesticide formulation—relation to safety in use. *J. Agr. Food Chem.*, **1**, 466–469.

Hazleton, L. W. and Holland, E. G. (1953). Toxicity of malathion. *Arch. industr. Hyg. Occup. Med.*, **8**, 399–405.

Healy, J. K. (1959). Ascending paralysis following malathion intoxication: A case report. *Med. J. Austr.*, **1**, 765–767.

Hearn, C. E. D. (1973). A review of agricultural pesticide incidents in man in England and Wales 1952–1971. *Brit. J. industr. Med.*, **30**, 253–258.

Heath, D. F. and Vandekar, M. (1957). Some spontaneous reactions of O,O-dimethyl S-ethylthioethyl phosphorothiolate and related compounds in water and on storage and their effects on the toxicological properties of the compounds. *Biochem. J.*, **67**, 187–201.

Heath, D. F. and Vandekar, M. (1964). Toxicity and metabolism of dieldrin in rats. *Brit. J. industr. Med.*, **21**, 269–279.

Hegazy, M. R. (1965). Poisoning by meta-isosystox in spraymen and in accidentally exposed patients. *Brit. J. industr. Med.*, **22**, 230–235.

Hermann, E. R. (1967). Threshold prediction and characteristics of log-normal phenomena. *Environ. Res.*, **1**, 359–369.

Hermann, E. R. (1971). Thresholds in biophysical systems. *Arch. Environ. Hlth.*, **22**, 699–706.

Hewlett, P. S. (1960). Joint action of insecticides. *Advances in Pest Control Research*, **3**, 27–74.

Hewlett, P. S. (1969). Measurement of the potencies of drug mixtures. *Biometrics*, **25**, 477–487.

Hewlett, P. S. and Plackett, R. L. (1961). 'Models for quantal responses to mixtures of two drugs' in *Quantitative Methods in Pharmacology*. Editor: H. de Jonge. (North-Holland Publishing Co.—Amsterdam).

Hicks, R. M. (1966). The permeability of rat transitional epithelium: Keratinization and the barrier to water. *J. Cell Biol.*, **28**, 21–31.

Hicks, R. (1975). Lesions in the respiratory system. *J. Pharm.*, **215**, 578–581.

Higuchi, T. (1960). Physical chemical analyses of percutaneous absorption process from creams and ointments. *J. Soc. Cosmet. Chem.*, **11**, 85–97.

Higuchi, T. and Kinkel, A. W. (1965). 'An apparatus for vapor pressure measurement of slightly volatile solutes' in *Surface Effects in Detection*. Editors: Bregman and Davnieks. Macmillan—London.

Hilado, C. J. and Furst, A. (1978). Reproducibility of toxicity test data as a function of mouse strain, animal lot and operator. *J. Combust. Toxicol.*, **5**, 75–80.

Hilbery, A. D. R., Waite, P. R. and McKinnon, J. (1973). Accidental poisoning in animals. *Vet. Rec.*, **92**, 489.

Hill, R. N., Clemens, T. L., Liv, D. K., Vesell, E. S. and Johnson, W. D. (1975). Genetic control of chloroform toxicity in mice. *Science*, **190**, 159–161.

Hodge, H. C. (1965). The LD_{50} and its value. *Am. Perfumer. Cosmet.*, **80**, 57–60.

Hodge, H. and Sterner, J. H. (1949). Tabulation of toxicity classes. *Amer. industr. Hyg. Assoc. Quart.*, **10**, 93–96.

Holcslaw, T. L., Miya, T. S. and Bousquet, W. S. (1975). Circadian rhythms in drug action and drug metabolism in the mouse. *J. Pharmacol. exptl. Therap.*, **195**, 320–332.

Holden, A. V. (1973). 'Effects of pesticides on fish' in *Environmental Pollution by Pesticides*. Editor: C. A. Edwards. Plenum Press—London and N.Y.

Holliday, M. A., Potter, D., Jarrah, A. and Bearg, S. (1967). The relation of metabolic rate to body weight and organ size. *Pediat. Res.*, **1**, 185–195.

Holmstedt, B. (1959). Pharmacology of organophosphorus cholinesterase inhibitors. *Pharmacol. Revs.*, **11**, 567–688.

Holtz, P. and Westerman, E. O. (1959). Toxicity and detoxification of parathion and paraoxon. (in German). *Nauryn—Schmiedebergs Arch. Pharmakol.*, **237**, 211–221.

Hommes, F. A. and Wilmink, C. W. (1968). Development changes of glycolytic enzymes in rat brain, liver and skeletal muscle. *Biol. Neonat.*, **12**, 181–193.

Hörnicke, H. (1977). Some characteristics of the digestive physiology of the rabbit. *ICLA Bulletin*, No. 41, 11–17.

136

Houston, J. B., Upshall, D. G. and Bridges, J. W. (1974). The re-evaluation of the importance of partition coefficients in the gastrointestinal absorption of anutrients. *J. Pharmacol. exptl. Ther.*, **189**, 244–254.

Houston, J. B., Upshall, D. G. and Bridges, J. W. (1975). Further studies using carbamate esters as model compounds to investigate the role of lipophilicity in the gastrointestinal absorption of foreign compounds. *J. Pharmacol. exptl Ther.*, **195**, 67–72.

Howard, W. E., Pacmateer, S. D. and Nachman, M. (1968). Aversion to strychnine sulfate by Norway rats, roof rats and pocket gophers. *Tox. Appl. Pharmacol.*, **12**, 229–241.

Hubble, D. R. and Taylor, A. T. (1976). The prolific Chinese hamster (*Cricetulus griseus*). *J. Inst. Anim. Tech.*, **27**, 100–107.

Hudson, D. R., Bass, G. E. and Purcell, W. P. (1970). Quantitative structure-activity models: Some conditions for application and statistical interpretation. *J. Med. Chem.*, **13**, 1184–1189.

Hudson, R. H., Tucker, R. K. and Haegece, M. A. (1972). Effect of age on sensitivity: Acute oral toxicity of 14 pesticides to Mallard ducks of several ages. *Tox. Appl. Pharmacol.*, **22**, 556–561.

Hughes, J. S. and Davis, J. T. (1963). Variations in toxicity to bluegill sunfish of phenoxy herbicides. *Weeds*, **11**, 50–53.

Hunt, J. N. (1963). Gastric emptying in relation to drug absorption. *Amer. J. Digest. Dis.*, **8**, 885–894.

Hunter, C. G. (1969). Dermal toxicity of chlorfenvinphos. *Industr. Med. Surg.*, **38**, 49–51.

Hunter, W. J. and Smeets, J. (1976). 'Acute Toxicity' in *The Evaluation of Toxicological Data for the Protection of Public Health*. Commission of the European Committees. Pergamon Press—Oxford.

Hurlbert, S. H. (1975). Secondary effects of pesticides on aquatic ecosystems. *Residue Revs.*, **57**, 81–148.

Hurst, E. W. (1958). 'Sexual differences in the toxicity and therapeutic action of chemical substances' in *The Evaluation of Drug Toxicity*. Editors: A. C. Walpole and A. Spinks. Little, Brown & Co.—Boston.

Hutson, D. H. and Hathway, D. E. (1967). Toxic effects of chlorfenvinphos in dogs and rats. *Biochem. Pharmacol.*, **16**, 949–962.

Hwang, S. W. and Schanker, L. S. (1973). Absorption of organic arsenic compounds from the rat small intestine. *Xenobiotica*, **3**, 351–355.

Hwang, S. W. and Schanker, L. S. (1974). Absorption of carbaryl from the lung and small intestine of the rat. *Environ. Res.*, **7**, 206–211.

Idson, B. (1971). 'Percutaneous absorption' in *Absorption Phenomena*. Editors: Rabinowitz and Myerson, Wiley–Interscience, New York and London.

Idson, B. (1975). Percutaneous absorption. *J. Pharm. Sci.*, **64**, 901–924.

Iunin, A. N. (1957). Speed and duration of sulphur-35 penetration through animal skin (in Russian). *Biul. Uses Inst. Vet. Sanitar.*, **2**, 11–12.

Ivey, M. C., Mann, H. D., Oehler, D. D., Claborn, H. V., Eschle, J. L. and Hogan, B. F. (1972). Chlorpyrifos and its oxygen analogue: Residues in the body tissues of dipped cattle. *J. Econ. Entomol.*, **65**, 1647–1649.

Jacobsen, P. L., Spear, R. C. and Wei, E. (1973). Parathion and diisopropylfluorophosphate (DFP) toxicity in partially hepatomized rats. *Tox. Appl. Pharmacol.*, **26**, 314–317.

Jager, K. W. (1970). *Aldrin, Dieldrin, Endrin and Telodrin*. Elsevier—Amsterdam.

Jager, K. W., Roberts, D. V. and Wilson, A. (1970). Neuromuscular function in pesticide workers. *Br. J. industr. Med.*, **27**, 273–278.

Jalili, M. A. and Abbasi, A. H. (1961). Poisoning by ethyl mercury toluene sulphonanilide. *Br. J. industr. Med.*, **18**, 303–308.

James, T. C. and Kanungo, M. S. (1976). Alterations in atropine sites of the brain of rats as a function of age. *Biochem. Biophys. Res. Commun.*, **72**, 170–175.

Janku, I. (1973). 'Problems in the evaluation of the relative biological potency of chemical agents', in *Adverse Effects of Environmental Chemicals and Psychotropic Drugs* Vol. 1. Editor: M. Horvath. Elsevier—Amsterdam, London and New York.

Janku, I. and Farghalli, H. M. (1971). Theoretische Beziehurgen zurischen akuter Toxizitat und pharmakokinetischen Konstanten. *Deutsche Apotheker—Zeitung*, **111**, 346.

Janku, I., Elis, J. and Raskova, H. (1971). Time–response curves in the evaluation of the clinical efficacy of drugs. *Europ. J. clin. Pharmacol.*, **3**, 194–197.

Jenkins, L. J., Jones, R. A. and Anderson, M. E. (1976). The use of mean survival time analysis in assessing toxic interactions. *Tox. Appl. Pharmacol.*, **37**, 129–130.

Jennings, D. M., Bunyan, P. J., Brown, P. M., Stanley, P. I. and Jones, F. J. S. (1975). Organophosphorus poisoning: A comparative study of the toxicity of carbophenothion to the Canada goose pigeon and Japanese quail. *Pestic. Sci.*, **6**, 245–257.

Jensen, A. L. (1972). Standard error of LC_{50} and sample size in fish bioassays. *Water Res.*, **6**, 85–89.

Johnson, H. D. and Voss, E. (1952). Toxicological studies of zinc phosphide. *J. Am. Pharm. Assoc. (Sci. Ed.)*, **41**, 468–472.

Johnson, J. H., Younger, R. L., Witzel, D. A. and Radeleff, R. D. (1975). Acute toxicity of tricyclohexyltin hydroxide to livestock. *Tox. Appl. Pharmacol.*, **31**, 66–71.

Johnston, B. L. and Eden, W. G. (1953). The toxicity of aldrin, dieldrin and toxaphene to rabbits by skin absorption. *J. Econ. Entomol.*, **46**, 702–703.

Jolly, D. W. (1970). 'Husbandry and Health of larger experimental animals' in *Nutrition and Disease in Experimental Animals*. Editor: W. D. Tavernor. Bailliere, Tindall and Cassell—London.

Jondorf, W. R., Maickel, R. P. and Brodie, T. M. (1958). Inability of newborn mice and guinea pigs to metabolize drugs. *Biochem. Pharmacol.*, **1**, 352–404.

Jones, C. J. (1978). The ranking of hazardous materials by means of hazard indices. *J. Hazard Mats.*, **2**, 263–289.

Jones, D. M. (1977). The occurrence of dieldrin in sawdust used as a bedding material. *Lab. Anim.*, **11**, 137.

Jordi, A. U. (1953). Absorption of methyl bromide through the intact skin. *J. Aviat. Med.*, **24**, 536–539.

Jori, A., Di Salle, E. and Santini, V. (1971). Daily rhythmic variation and liver drug metabolism in rats. *Biochem. Pharmacol.*, **20**, 2965–2969.

Jovic, R. C. (1974). Correlation between signs of toxicity and some biochemical changes in rats poisoned by Soman. *Eur. J. Pharmacol.*, **25**, 159–164.

Kakemi, K., Sezaki, H., Konishi, R., Kimura, T. and Murakami, M. (1970). Effect of bile salts on the gastro-intestinal absorption of drugs. *Chem. Pharm. Bull.*, **18**, 275–280.

Kalow, W. (1962). *Pharmacogenetics—Heredity and the Response to Drugs*. W. B. Saunders, Co., Philadelphia and London.

Kalow, W. (1965). Dose–response relationship and genetic variation. *Ann. N.Y. Acad. Sci.*, **123**, 212–218.

Kaloyanova-Simeonova, F. and Fournier, E. (1971). *Les pesticides et l'homme*. Masson et Cie—Paris.

Kaminski, M. (1964). Esterases in avian sera: Species specific pattern and individual variation. *Experientia*, **20**, 286–287.

Kaplan, H. M. and Overpeck, J. G. (1964). Toxicity of halogenated hydrocarbon insecticides for the frog. *Rana pipiens. Herpetologica*, **20**, 163–169.

Kärber, G. (1931). Beitrog zur Kollektiven Behandlung pharmakologischer Reihenversuche. *Arch. exptl Path. Pharmakol.*, **162**, 480–483.

Kastin, A. J., Arimura, A. and Schally, A. V. (1966). Topical absorption of polypeptides with dimethylsulfoxide. *Arch. Derm.*, **93**, 471–473.

Kato, R. (1974). Sex-related differences in drug metabolism. *Drug Metabol. Rev.*, **3**, 1–32.

Kato, R. and Gillette, J. R. (1965). Sex differences in the effects of abnormal physiological states on the metabolism of drugs by rat liver microsomes. *J. Pharmacol. exptl. Ther.*, **150**, 285–291.

Kato, R. and Onoda, K. (1966). Effect of morphine administration on the activity of microsomal drug-metabolizing enzyme systems in liver of different species. *Jap. J. Pharmacol.*, **16**, 217–219.

Kato, R., Onoda, K. and Takanaka, A. (1971). Species differences in the effect of morphine administration or adrenalectomy on the substrate interaction with cytochrome P-450 and drug oxidations by liver microsomes. *Biochem. Pharmacol.*, **20**, 1093–1099.

Kato, R., Vassanelli, P., Frontino, G. and Chiesara, E. (1964). Variation in the activity of liver microsomal drug-metabolizing enzymes in rats in relation to the age. *Biochem. Pharmacol.*, **13**, 1037–1051.

Katz, M. and Poulsen, B. J. (1971). 'Absorption of drugs through the skin' in *Concepts of Biochemical Pharmacology*. Vol. 28. Editors: R. B. Brodie and J. R. Gillette. Springer-Verlag—Berlin, Heidelberg and N.Y.

Katz, M. and Shaikh, Z. I. (1965). Percutaneous corticosteroid absorption correlated to partition coefficient. *J. Pharm. Sci.*, **54**, 591–594.

138

Kazantzis, G., McLaughlin, A. I. G. and Prior, P. F. (1964). Poisoning in industrial workers by the insecticide aldrin. *Brit. J. industr. Med.*, **21**, 46–51.

Keberle, H. (1971). Physico-chemical factors of drugs affecting absorption, distribution and excretion. *Acta Pharmacol. Toxicol.*, **29**, (Supp. 3), 30–47.

Kedem, O. and Katchalsky, A. (1961). A physical interpretation of the phenomenological coefficients of membrane permeability. *J. Gen. Physiol.*, **45**, 143–179.

Kelsey, F. (1971). Poisoning from insecticides. *Vet. Rec.*, **88**, 136.

Keplinger, M. L. and Deichmann, W. B. (1967). Acute toxicity of combinations of pesticides. *Tox. Appl. Pharmacol.*, **10**, 586–595.

Keplinger, M. L., Lanier, G. E. and Deichmann, W. B. (1959). Effects of environmental temperature on the acute toxicity of a number of compounds in rats. *Tox. Appl. Pharmacol.*, **1**, 156–161.

Khan, M. A. (1973). Toxicity of systemic insecticides: Toxicological considerations in using organophosphorus insecticides. *Vet. Rec.*, **92**, 411–418.

Khan, M. A. and Haufe, W. O. (1972). (Editors) *Toxicology Biodegradation and Efficacy of Livestock Pesticides*. Swets and Zeitlinger—Amsterdam.

Khan, M. A. Q., Khan, H. M. and Sutherland, D. J. (1973). 'Ecological and health effects of the photolysis of insecticides' in *Survival in Toxic Environments*. Editors: M. A. Q. Khan and J. P. Bederka, Jr.

Khera, K. S. and Clegg, D. J. (1969). Perinatal toxicity of pesticides. *Canad. Med. Assoc. J.*, **100**, 167–172.

Kimbrough, R. D. (1976). Toxicity and health effects of selected organotin compounds: A review. *Environ. Hlth. Perspect.*, **14**, 51–56.

Kimbrough, R. D., Carter, C. D., Liddle, J. A., Cline, R. E. and Phillips, P. E. (1977). Epidemiology and pathology of a tetrachlorodibenzodioxin poisoning episode. *Arch. Environ. Hlth.*, **32**, 77–86.

Kimbrough, R. D. and Gaines, T. B. (1970). Toxicity of paraquat to rats and its effects on rats lungs. *Tox. Appl. Pharmacol.*, **17**, 679–690.

Kimmerle, G. and Lorke, D. (1968). Toxicology of insecticidal organophosphates. *Pflanzenschutz-Nachrichten Bayer*, **21**, 111–142.

Kimura, E. T., Elbert, D. M. and Dodge, P. W. (1971). Acute toxicity and limits of solvent residue for sixteen organic solvents. *Tox. Appl. Pharmacol.*, **19**, 699–704.

King, J. R. and Farner, D. S. (1961). 'Energy metabolism, thermoregulation and body temperature' in, *Biology and Comparative Physiology of Birds*. Editor: A. J. Marshall. Academic Press—N.Y. and London.

King, E. and Harvey, D. G. (1953). Some observations on the absorption and excretion of 4,6-dinitro-*o*-cresol (DNOC). *Biochem. J.*, **53**, 185–200.

Kleiber, M. (1975). Metabolic tumour rate: A physiological meaning of the metabolic rate per unit body weight. *J. theor. Biol.*, **53**, 199–204.

Klemmer, H. W. (1972). Human health and pesticides—community pesticide studies. *Residue Rev.*, **41**, 55–61.

Klevay, L. M. (1970). Dieldrin excretion by the isolated perfused rat liver: A sexual difference. *Tox. Appl. Pharmacol.*, **17**, 813–815.

Kling, T. G. and Long, K. R. (1969). Blood cholinesterase in previously stressed animals subjected to parathion. *J. Occup. Med.*, **11**, 82–84.

Kloche, R. A., Gurtner, G. H. and Farhe, L. E. (1963). Gas transfer across the skin in man. *J. Appl. Physiol.*, **18**, 311–316.

Knaak, J. B. and O'Brien, R. D. (1960). Effect of EPN on *in vivo* metabolism of malathion by the rat and dog. *J. Agr. Food Chem.*, **8**, 198–203.

Knudsen, L. F. and Curtis, J. M. (1947). The use of angular transformation in biological assays. *J. Amer. Statist. Assoc.*, **42**, 282–296.

Koch, A. L. (1966). The logarithm in biology: I. Mechanisms generating the log-normal distribution exactly. *J. theor. Biol.*, **12**, 276–290.

Koch, A. L. (1969). The logarithm in biology: II. Distributions simulating the log-normal. *J. theor. Biol.*, **23**, 251–268.

Kocsis, J. J., Harkaway, S. and Snyder, R. (1968). Potentiating effect of dimethyl sulphoxide in toxicity of various solvent hydrocarbons. *Pharmacologist*, **10**, 72.

Koeffler, H. (1958). Akute E-605-Vergiftung durch percutane Giftaufrahme. *Med. Klin.*, **53**, 749–751.

Kondritzer, A. A., Mayer, W. H. and Zvirblis, P. (1959). Removal of sarin from skin and eyes. *Arch. industr. Hlth.*, **20**, 50–52.

139

Krasner, J. (1973). Theoretical considerations of drug–protein binding. *Rev. Com. Biol.*, **32** (Suppl.), 133–134.

Krasovskij, G. N. (1975). 'Species and sex differences in sensitivity to toxic substances' in, *Methods used in the USSR for Establishing Biologically Safe Levels of Toxic Substances*. Wld. Hlth. Org.,—Geneva.

Krasovskij, G. N. (1976). Extrapolation of experimental data from animals to man. *Environ. Hlth. Perspect.*, **13**, 51–58.

Krebs, H. A. (1950). Body size and tissue respiration. *Biochem. Biophys. Acta*, **4**, 249–269.

Krijnen, C. J. and Boyd, E. M. (1971). The influence of diets containing from 0 to 81% of protein on tolerated doses of pesticides. *Comp. gen. Pharmac.*, **2**, 373–376.

Kruger, S., Greve, D. W. and Schueler, F. W. (1962). The absorption of fluid from the peritoneal cavity. *Arch. int. Pharmacodyn.*, **137**, 173–178.

Kuchmeister, H., Pliess, G. and Wilhelm, W. (1955). Untersuchungen uber die Fraktimierte schadigung der nebennieren-rinde des Hundes mit 2,2-bis(p-chlorophenyl)-1 : 1-dichloro-ethane (DDD). *Acta Endocrin.*, **20**, 39–46.

Kundiev, Y. I. (1963). On the absorption through the skin of thiophosphoric acid esters series (in Russian). *Farmakol. Toksikol.*, **26**, 361–365.

Kundiev, Y. I. (1965). Effect of some organophosphorus insecticides which gain access through the skin (in Russian). *Farmakol. Tokiskol.*, **28**, 238–241.

Kupferberg, H. J. and Way, E. L. (1963). Pharmacologic basis for the increased sensitivity of the new-born rat to morphine. *J. Pharmacol. exptl. Ther.*, **141**, 105–112.

Kurtz, P. J. (1977). Dissociated behavioral and cholinesterase decrements following malathion exposure. *Tox. Appl. Pharmacol.*, **42**, 589–594.

Lakota, S. (1974). Attempt to classify pesticides according to toxicity for freshwater fish (in Polish). *Gaz. Woda Tech. Sorit.*, **48**, 270–271. (*Pesticide Abstracts* 1975, 75-0377).

Lamanna, C. and Hart, E. R. (1968). Relationship of lethal toxic dose to body weight of the mouse. *Tox. Appl. Pharmacol.*, **13**, 307–315.

Landahl, H. D. (1958). Theoretical considerations on potentiation in drug interaction. *Bull. Math. Biophys.*, **20**, 1–23.

Lang, C. M. and Vessell, E. S. (1976). Environmental and genetic factors affecting laboratory animals: Impact on biomedical research. *Fed. Proc.*, **35**, 1123–1124.

Lanman, R. C., Stremsterfer, C. E. and Schanker, L. S. (1971). Absorption of organic anions from the rat small intestine. *Xenobiotica*, **1**, 613–619.

Laroche, M. J. (1965). Influence of environment on drug activity in laboratory animals. *Fd Cosmet. Toxicol.*, **3**, 177–191.

Lasagna, L. (1956). Drug effects as modified by aging. *J. Chron. Dis.*, **3**, 567–574.

Lautenschläger, J., Grabensee, B. and Pottgen, W. (1974). Paraquat intoxication und isolierte Aplastische Anamie. *Dtsch med. Wschr.*, **99**, 2348–2351.

Laws, E. R., Curley, A. and Biros, F. J. (1967). Men with intensive occupational exposure to DDT. *Arch. Environ. Health*, **15**, 766–775.

Lee, M. M. C. and Ng, C. K. (1965). Postmortem studies of skinfold caliper measurement and actual thickness of skin and subcutaneous tissue. *Human Biol.*, **37**, 91–103.

Lee, R. M. (1964). Di-(2-chloroethyl)-aryl phosphates: A study of their reaction with β-esterases and of the genetic control of their hydrolysis in sheep. *Biochem. Pharmacol.*, **13**, 1551–1568.

Lee, R. M. and Pickering, W. R. (1967). The toxicity of haloxon to geese, ducks and hens, and its relationship to the stability of the di-(2-chloroethyl)phosphoryl cholinesterase derivatives. *Biochem. Pharmacol.*, **16**, 941–948.

Lees, P. (1972). Pharmacology and toxicology of alphachloralose: A review. *Vet. Rec.*, **91**, 320–333.

Lehman, A. J. (1959). 'Some relations of drug toxicity in experimental animals compared to man' in, *Appraisal of Safety of Chemicals in Foods, Drugs and Cosmetics*. Editors: Staff of Division of Pharmacology of Food and Drug Administration, U.S. Dept. of Health, Education and Welfare. Association of Food and Drug Officials of the United States.

Leider, M. and Buncke, C. M. (1954). Physical dimensions of the skin. *Arch. Derm. Syph.*, **69**, 563–569.

Lenox, R. H. and Frazier, T. W. (1972). Methadone induced mortality as a function of the circadian cycle. *Nature*, **239**, 397–398.

Lesser, G. T., Deutsch, S. and Markofsky, J. (1973). Aging in the rat: Longitudinal and cross-sectional studies of body composition. *Am. J. Physiol.*, **225**, 1472–1478.

140

Leuzinger, S., Pasi, A. and Dolder, R. (1971). Synoptical review of 536 cases of alkylphosphate poisoning (in German). *Schweiz. Med. Wschr.*, **101**, 563–570.

Levin, H. S. (1974). 'Behavioral effects of occupational exposure to organophosphate pesticides' in *Behavioral Toxicology*. Editors: C. Xintoras, B. L. Johnson and I. de Groot. U.S. Dept. of Health, Education and Welfare, Public Health Service Center for Disease Control, N.I.O.S.H.—Washington, D.C.

Levin, H. S. and Rodnitzky, R. L. (1976). Behavioral effects of organophosphate pesticides in man. *Clin. Toxicol.*, **9**, 391–405.

Levitsky, D. A. and Barnes, R. G. (1972). Nutritional and environmental interactions in the behavioral developments of the rat. *Science*, **176**, 68–71.

Lewin, J. F. and Love, J. L. (1974). A death caused by the ingestion of mevinphos. *Forensic Sci.*, **4**, 253–255.

Lien, E. J. and Tong, G. L. (1973). Physiochemical properties and percutaneous absorption of drugs. *J. Soc. Cosmet. Chem.*, **24**, 371–384.

Lien, E., Koda, R. T. and Tong, G. L. (1971). Buccal and percutaneous absorptions. *Drug Intel. Clin. Pharm.*, **5**, 38–41.

Lindsey, D. (1962). Percutaneous penetration. *Proc. Int. Congr. Dermatol.*—Washington, D.C.

Lisella, F. S. (1972). Epidemiology of poisoning by chemicals. *J. environ. Hlth.*, **34**, 603–612.

Litchfield, J. T. (1967). Drug toxicity in the human fetus and newborn child. *Appl. Therap.*, **9**, 922–926.

Litchfield, J. T. and Wilcoxon, F. (1949). A simplified method of evaluating dose–effect experiments. *J. Pharmacol. exptl. Ther.*, **96**, 99–115.

Litchfield, M. H., Daniel, J. W. and Longshaw, S. (1973). The tissue distribution of the bipyridylium herbicide diquat and paraquat in rats and mice. *Toxicology*, **1**, 155–165.

Litterst, C. L., Mimnaugh, F. G., Regan, R. L. and Gram, T. E. (1975). Comparison of *in vitro* drug metabolism by lung, liver and kidney of several common laboratory species. *Drug Metab. Dispos.*, **3**, 259–265.

Ljublina, E. I. and Filov, V. A. (1975). 'Chemical structure, physical and chemical properties and biological activity' in, *Methods Used in the USSR for Establishing Biologically Safe Levels of Toxic Substances*. Wld. Hlth. Org.—Geneva.

Ljublina, E. I. and Rabotnikova, L. V. (1970). The possibility of pre-determining the toxicities of volatile organic compounds from their physical constants (in Russian). *Gig. Sanit.*, **36**, 33–37.

Lloyd, G. A. and Bell, G. J. (1967). The exposure of agricultural workers to pesticides used in granular form. *Ann. Occup. Hyg.*, **10**, 97–104.

Lloyd, T. S. (1973). Accidental poisoning in birds. *Vet. Rec.*, **92**, 489.

Locati, G., Cavagna, G. and Bugatti, A. (1968). Study on the penetration of phosdrin through protective gloves. *Med. Lavora*, **59**, 342–345.

Loeb, H. A. and Engstrom-Heg, R. (1970). Time dependent changes in toxicity of rotenone dispersions to trout. *Tox. Appl. Pharmacol.*, **17**, 605–614.

Loewe, S. (1938). Coalitive actions of combined drugs. *J. Pharmacol. exptl. Ther.*, **63**, 24.

Long, K. R. (1975). Cholinesterase activity as a biological indicator of exposure to pesticides. *Int. Arch. Occup. Environ. Hlth.*, **36**, 75–86.

Lovejoy, G. S. (1975). Quoted in *Local Tennessee Health Dept. Submits Report on Arsenic Poisoning History*. Pesticide Chemical New, **3**, 21–22.

Lowrance, W. W. (1976). *Of Acceptable Risk*. William Kaufmann, Inc.—Los Altos, Calif.

Lu, F. C., Jessup, D. C. and Lavallee, A. (1965). Toxicity of pesticides in young versus adult rats. *Fd Cosmet. Toxicol.*, **3**, 591–596.

Luckey, T. D. and Venugopal, B. (1977). pT, a new classification system for toxic chemicals. *J. Toxicol. environ. Hlth.*, **2**, 633–638.

Luckmann, W. H. and Decker, G. C. (1960). A 5-year report of observations in the Japanese beetle control area at Sheldon, Illinois. *J. Econ. Entomol.*, **53**, 821–827.

Lueck, L. M., Wurster, D. E., Higuchi, T., Finger, K. F., Lemberger, A. P. and Busse, L. W. (1957a). Investigation and development of protective ointments: I. Development of a method for measuring permeation of mechanical barriers. *J. Am. Pharm.Assoc. (Sci. Ed.)*, **46**, 694–697.

Lueck, L. M., Wurster, D. E., Higuchi, T., Finger, K. F., Lemberger, A. P. and Busse, L. W. (1957b). Investigation and development of protective ointments: II. Influence of partition coefficients and thickness. *J. Am. Pharm. Assoc. (Sci. Ed)*, **46**, 698–701.

Lukas, G., Brindle, S. D. and Greengard, P. (1971). The route of absorption of intraperitoneally administered compounds. *J. Pharmacol. exptl. Ther.*, **178**, 562–566.

Lynch, W. T. and Coon, J. M. (1972). Effect of tri-*o*-tolyl phosphate pretreatment on the toxicity and metabolism of parathion and paraoxon in mice. *Tox. Appl. Pharmacol.*, **21**, 153–165.

McArthur, J. N., Dawkins, P. D. and Smith, M. J. H. (1971). Of mice and means. *Nature*, **229**, 66.

McCreesh, A. H. (1965). Percutaneous toxicity. *Tox. Appl. Pharmacol.*, **7**, (Supp. 2), 20–26.

McDonaugh, B. J. and Martin, J. (1970). Paraquat poisoning in children. *Arch. Dis. Child.*, **45**, 425–427.

McElligott, T. F. (1972). The dermal toxicity of paraquat: Differences due to techniques of application. *Tox. Appl. Pharmacol.*, **21**, 361–368.

McFarland, L. Z. and Lacey, P. B. (1968). Acute anticholinesterases toxicity in ducks and Japanese quail. *Tox. Appl. Pharmacol.*, **12**, 105–114.

McLean, A. E. M. (1971). 'Conversion by the liver of inactive molecules into toxic molecules' in *Mechanisms of Toxicity*. Editor: W. N. Aldridge. Macmillan—London.

McLeod, W. R. (1975). Merphos poisoning or mass panic. *Aust. N.Z.J. Psychiatry*, **9**, 225–229.

McPhail, M. K. and Adie, P. A. (1960). Penetration of radioactive isopropyl methylphosphonofluoridate (Sarin) vapor through skin. *Can. J. Biochem. Physiol.*, **38**, 935–944.

McPhillips, J. J. (1969). Altered sensitivity to drugs following repeated injection of a cholinesterase inhibitor to rats. *Tox. Appl. Pharmacol.*, **14**, 67–73.

McSmith, W. and Ledbetter, J. O. (1971). Hazards from fires involving organophosphorus insecticides. *Amer. industr. Hyg. Assoc. J.*, **32**, 468–474.

Macek, K. J., Hutchinson, C. and Cope, O. B. (1969). The effects of temperature on the susceptibility of bluegills and rainbow trout to selected pesticides. *Bull. environ. Contam. Toxicol.*, **4**, 174–179.

MacFarland, H. N. (1975). Inhalation toxicology. *J.A.O.A.C.*, **58**, 689–691.

Machin, A. F., Anderson, P. H. and Herbert, C. N. (1974). Residue levels and cholinesterase activities in sheep poisoned experimentally with diazinon. *Pestic. Sci.*, **5**, 49–56.

Maeda, T., Takenaka, H., Yamahira, Y. and Noguchi, T. (1977). Use of rabbits for GI drug absorption studies. *J. Pharm. Sci.*, **66**, 69–73.

Magalhaes, H. (1968). 'Gross Anatomy' in, *The Golden Hamster: its Biology and Use in Medical Research*. Editors: R. A. Hoffman, P. E. Robinson and H. Magalhees. Iowa State University Press—Ames, Iowa.

Maibach, H. J., Feldmann, R., Milby, T. and Serat, W. (1970). Percutaneous penetration of pesticides in man—a preliminary report. *Proceedings Symposium Sulla Prevenzione Dermatosi Professionali*, (Monte Porzio Catone).

Maibach, H. I., Feldmann, R. J., Milby, T. and Serat, W. F. (1971). Regional variation in percutaneous penetration in man. *Arch. environ. Hlth.*, **23**, 208–211.

Maines, M. D. and Westfall, B. A. (1971). Sex difference in the metabolism of hexobarbitone in the Mongolian gerbil. *Proc. Soc. Exp. Biol. Med.*, **138**, 820–822.

Majda, A. (1976). Optimalisation endeavour of the numerousness of animals in experimental groups in acute toxicity routine estimation assays on rats. *Zwierzete Lab.*, **13**, 37–45.

Majno, G. and Karnovsky, M. L. (1961). A biochemical and morphologic study of myelination and demyelination (III) Effect of an organophosphorus compound (MIPAFOX) on the biosynthesis of lipid by nervous tissue of rats and hens. *J. Neurochem.*, **8**, 1–16.

Mali, J. W. (1956). The transport of water through the human epidermis. *J. Invest. Derm.*, **27**, 451–469.

Malone, J. C. (1964). Toxicity of haloxon. *Res. Vet. Sci.*, **5**, 17–31.

Mancini, R. E. and Kocsis, J. J. (1974). Dimethylsulphoxide increases the lethality of CCl_4 in rats but decreases its hepatotoxicity. *Tox. Appl. Pharmacol.*, **27**, 206–209.

Mann, Jr., D. E. (1965). Biological aging and its modification of drug activity. *J. Pharm. Sci.*, **54**, 499–510.

Mant, A. K. (1960). *Forensic Medicine*. Lloyd-Luke—London.

Mark, L. C. (1971). 'Translocation of drugs and other exogenous chemicals into adipose tissue' in *Handbook of Experimental Pharmacology* Vol. 28 (Pt 1). Springer-Verlag—Berlin, Heidelberg, and N.Y.

Marliac, J. P., Verrett, M. J., McLaughlin, Jr., J. and Fitzhugh, O. H. (1965). A comparison of toxicity data obtained for twenty-one pesticides by the chicken embryo technique with acute oral LD_{50}'s in rats. (Abstract only). *Tox. Appl. Pharmacol.*, 7, 490 (only).

Marte, E. and Halberg, F. (1961). Circadian susceptibility rhythm of mice to librium. *Fed. Proc.*, 20, 305.

Martinez-O'Ferrall, J. A. (1968). Circadian rhythms. *J. Occup. Med.*, 10, 305–315.

Marzulli, F. N. (1962). Barriers to skin penetration. *J. Invest. Derm.*, 39, 387–393.

Marzulli, F. N. and Tregar, R. T. (1961). Identification of a barrier layer in the skin. *J. Physiol.*, 157, 52P.

Marzulli, F. N., Callaghan, J. F. and Brown, D. W. C. (1965). Chemical structure and skin penetrating capacity of a short series of organic phosphates and phosphoric acid. *J. Invest. Derm.*, 44, 339–344.

Mason, M. M. (1971). 'Toxicology of DMSO in animals' in *Dimethyl Sulphoxide*. Editors: S. W. Jacob, E. E. Rosenbaum and D. C. Wood. Marcel Dekker Inc.,—N.Y.

Masterson, J. G. and Roche, W. J. (1970). Another paraquat fatality. *Br. Med. J.*, ii, 5707.

Matsushima, S. and Abe, E. (1974). The effectiveness and limitations of simian animals in toxicity experiments (in Japanese). *Jikken Dobutsu*, 23, 272–273. (*Pestic. Abstr.* 75–1178).

Matthews, G. A. and Clayphon, J. E. (1973). Safety precautions for pesticide application in the tropics. *PANS*, 19, 1–12.

Mattock, G. L. and McGilveray, I. J. (1973). The effect of food intake and sleep on the absorption of acetamenophen. *Rev. Can. Biol.*, 32 (Suppl.), 77–84.

Mauck, W. L. and Olson, L. E. (1976). Toxicity of natural pyrethrins and five pyrethroids to fish. *Arch. environ. Contam.*, 4, 18–29.

Mawdesley-Thomas, L. E. (1971). Toxic chemicals—the risk to fish. *New Sci.*, 49, 74–75.

Mawdesley-Thomas, L. E., Jolley, D. W., Jenkins, G. and Bucke, D. (1974). The fish as a toxicological tool. *Tox. Appl. Pharmacol.*, 29, 111.

May, G. (1973). Chloracne from the accidental production of tetrachlorodibenzodioxin. *Brit. J. industr. Med.*, 3, 276–283.

Mayer, F. L., Street, J. C. and Neuhold, J. M. (1972). DDT intoxication in rainbow trout as affected by dieldrin. *Tox. Appl. Pharmacol.*, 22, 347–354.

Medved, L. I. and Kundiev, Y. I. (1964). On the methods of study of penetration of chemical substances through the intact skin (Russian). *Gig. Sanit.*, 29, 71–76.

Medved, L. I., Spynu, E. I. and Kagan, I. S. (1964). The method of conditioned reflexes in toxicology and its application for determining the toxicity of small quantities of pesticides. *Residue Revs.*, 6, 41–47.

Meeter, E. and Wolthuis, O. L. (1968a). The effects of cholinesterase inhibitors on the body temperature of the rat. *Europ. J. Pharmacol.*, 4, 18–24.

Meeter, E. and Wolthuis, O. L. (1968b). The spontaneous recovery of respiration and neuromuscular transmission in the rat after anticholinesterase poisoning. *Eur. J. Pharmacol.*, 2, 377–386.

Meeter, E., Wolthuis, O. L. and van Benthem, R. M. J. (1971). The anticholinesterase hypothermia in the rat: Its practical application in the study of the central effectiveness of oximes. *Bull. Wld. Hlth. Org.*, 44, 251–257.

Mehrle, P. M., Johnson, W. and Mayer, Jr., F. L. (1973). Quoted in *Use of Biological Tests for Evaluation of Pesticides* by E. E. Kenaga. *Pure and Appl. Chem.*, (1975), 42, 285–299.

Meier, H. (1963a). 'Potentialities for and present status of pharmacological research in genetically controlled mice' in *Advances in Pharmacology* Vol. 2. Editors: S. Garattini and P. A. Shore. Academic Press—N.Y. and London.

Meier, H. (1963b). *Experimental Pharmacogenetics: Physiopathology of Heredity and Pharmacologic Responses*. Academic Press—N.Y. and London.

Mellett, L. B. (1969). Comparative drug metabolism. *Proc. Drug Res.*, 13, 138–169.

Mendoza, C. E. and Shields, J. B. (1977). Effects on esterases and comparison of I_{50} and LD_{50} values of malathion in suckling rats. *Bull. Environ. Contam. Toxicol.*, 17, 9–15.

Menzer, R. E. (1970). Effect of chlorinated hydrocarbons in the diet on the toxicity of several organophosphorus insecticides. *Tox. Appl. Pharmacol.*, 16, 446–452.

Mercer, T. T. (1973). *Aerosol Technology in Hazard Evaluation*. Academic Press—N.Y. and London.

Mertens, H. W., Lewis, M. F. and Steen, J. A. (1974). Some behavioral effects of pesticides: Phosdrin and free-operant escape-avoidance behaviour in gerbils. *Aerosp. Med.*, 45, 1171–1176.

Mertens, H. W., Steen, J. A. and Lewis, M. F. (1975). The effects of mevinphos on appetitive operant behaviour in the gerbil. *Psychopharmacologica*, **41**, 47–52.

Metcalf, R. L. (1957). Control of hazards in use of agricultural chemicals—California experience. *AMA Arch. industr. Health*, **16**, 337–352.

Meyer, B. J. and Karel, L. (1948). The effect of environmental temperature of alphanaphthylthiourea toxicity to rats. *J. Pharmacol. exptl. Ther.*, **93**, 420–422.

Mia, A. S., Latif, A. and Ali, K. M. (1973). Comparative toxicity of certain organophosphorus insecticides in goat. *Bangladesh J. Biol. Agric. Sci.*, **2**, 17–19.

Miller, D. S., Stirling, J. L. and Yudkin, J. (1966). Effect of ingestion of milk on concentrations of blood alcohol. *Nature*, **212**, 1051.

Miller, L. C. (1964). 'The quantal response in toxicity tests' in *Statistics and Mathematics in Biology*. Editors: O. Kempthorne, T. A. Bancroft, J. W. Gowen and J. L. Lush. Hafner Publishing Co.—N.Y.

Miller, L. C. and Tainter, M. L. (1944). Estimation of the ED_{50} and its error by means of logarithmic probit graph paper. *Proc. Soc. Exp. Biol.*, **57**, 261–264.

Mitchell, E. W. and Schanker, L. S. (1973). Absorption of organic compounds from the mouse lung. *Fed. Proc.*, **32**, 258.

Miura, K., Ino, T. and Izuka, S. (1974). Comparison of the susceptibilities to the acute toxicity of BHC in strains of experimental mice (in Japanese). *Jikken Dobutsu*, **2**, 198.

Moffat, A. C. (1971). 'Absorption of Drugs Through the Oral Mucosa' in *Absorption Phenomena*. Editors: J. Rabinowitz and R. Myerson. Wiley–Interscience—New York and London.

Moore, D. H. (1972). 'Species, Sex and Strain Differences in Metabolism' in *Foreign Compound Metabolism in Mammals*. Editor: D. E. Hathway. The Chemical Society—London.

Morello, A., Spencer, A. Y. and Vardanis, A. (1967). Biochemical mechanisms in the toxicity of the geometrical isomers of two vinyl organophosphates. *Biochem. Pharmacol.*, **16**, 1703–1710.

Morello, A., Vardanis, A. and Spencer, A. Y. (1968). Comparative metabolism of two vinyl phosphorothionate isomers (thiono-Phosdrin) by the mouse and the fly. *Biochem. Pharmacol.*, **17**, 1795–1802.

Moriyama, I., Ichikawa, H. and Ide, H. (1972). Death after accidental ingestion of Gramoxone resulting in fibrosis of the lung (in Japanese). *Nippon Noson Igakkai Zasshi.*, **21**, 244–245.

Mörnstad, H. (1975). Acute sodium fluoride toxicity in rats in relation to age and sex. *Acta pharmacol. Toxicol.*, **37**, 425–428.

Morrow, P. E. (1960). Some physical and physiological factors controlling the fate of inhaled substances. *Health Physics.*, **2**, 366–378.

Muirhead-Thomson, R. C. (1971). *Pesticides and Freshwater Fauna*. Academic Press—London and N.Y.

Muller, P. J. and Vernikos-Danellis, J. (1968). Alteration in drug toxicity by environmental variables. *Proc. Western Pharmacol. Soc.*, **11**, 52–53.

Mullins, L. J. (1954). Some physical mechanisms in narcosis. *Chem. Rev.*, **54**, 289–323.

Munoz-Villegas, M. and Carcur-Giacaman, C. (1971). Organophosphate pesticide poisoning in children (in Spanish). *Rev. Chil. Pediat.*, **42**, 361–364.

Munro, I. B., Ostler, D. C., Machin, A. F. and Quick, M. P. (1977). Suspected poisoning by pentachlorophenol in sawdust. *Vet. Rec.*, **101**, 525 (only).

Murphy, P. G. (1971). The effect of size on the uptake of DDT from water by fish. *Bull. environ. Contam. Tox.*, **6**, 20–23.

Murphy, S. D. (1969a). Some relationships between effects of insecticides and other stress conditions. *Ann. N.Y. Acad. Sci.*, **160**, 366–377.

Murphy, S. D. (1969b). Mechanisms of pesticide interactions in vertebrates. *Residue Reviews*, **25**, 201–221.

Murphy, S. D. and Cheever, K. L. (1972). Carboxylesterase and cholinesterase inhibition in rats. *Arch. environ. Hlth.*, **24**, 107–114.

Murphy, S. D. and Dubois, K. P. (1958). Inhibitory effect of dipterex and other organic phosphates on detoxification of malathion. *Federation Proc.*, **17**, 397.

Murphy, S. D., Anderson, R. L. and Dubois, K. P. (1959). Potentiation of toxicity of malathion by triorthotolylphosphate. *Proc. Soc. exptl. Biol. Med.*, **100**, 483–487.

Murphy, S. D., Lauwerys, R. R. and Cheever, K. L. (1968). Comparative anticholinesterase

144

action of organophosphorus insecticides in vertebrates. *Tox. Appl. Pharmacol.*, **12**, 22–35.

Murray, R. E. and Gibson, J. E. (1972). A comparative study of paraquat intoxication in rats, guinea pigs and monkeys. *Exptl. Mol. Path.*, **17**, 317–325.

Murray, R. E. and Gibson, J. E. (1974). Paraquat disposition in rats, guinea pigs and monkeys. *Tox. Appl. Pharmacol.*, **27**, 283–291.

Myers, K. (1976). Further observations on the 'TARBABY' technique for poisoning rabbits. *Int. Pest. Contr.*, **18**, 10–17.

Nabb, D. P., Stein, W. J. and Hayes, Jr., W. J. (1966). Rate of skin absorption of parathion and paraoxon. *Arch. environ. Hlth.*, **12**, 501–505.

Nagata, H. (1972). On the recent health conditions of pesticide speed sprayers (in Japanese). *Nippon Noson Igakkai Zosshi*, **21**, 232–233.

Naik, S. R., Anjaria, R. J. and Sheth, U. K. (1970). Studies on rat brain acetylcholine and cholinesterase, Pt 1. Effect of body weight, sex, stress and CNS depressant drugs. *Indian J. Med. Res.*, **58**, 473–479.

Namba, T. (1971). Cholinesterase inhibition by organophosphorus compounds and its clinical effects. *Bull. Wld. Hlth. Org.*, **44**, 289–307.

Namba, T., Nolte, C. T., Jackrel, J. and Grob, D. (1971). Poisoning due to organophosphate insecticides: Acute and chronic manifestations. *Am. J. Med.*, **50**, 475–492.

National Academy of Sciences (Washington D.C.) (1971). 'Defining the laboratory animal'. *Proceedings of 4th Symposium of the International Committee on Laboratory Animals.*

Natoff, I. L. (1967). Influence of the route of administration on the toxicity of some cholinesterase inhibitors. *J. Pharm. Pharmac.*, **19**, 612–616.

Natoff, I. L. (1973). 'The importance of dose–response parameters in acute toxicity studies' in *Adverse Effects of Environmental Chemicals and Psychotrophic Drugs* Vol. 1. Editor: M. Horvath. Elsevier—Amsterdam, London, New York.

Natoff, I. L. and Reiff, B. (1970). Quantitative studies on the effect of antagonists on the acute toxicity of organophosphates in rats. *Br. J. Pharmac.*, **40**, 124–134.

Neal, R. A. (1972). A comparison of the *in vitro* metabolism of parathion in the lung and liver of the rabbit. *Tox. Appl. Pharmacol.*, **23**, 123–130.

Neely, W. A., Turner, M. D. and Taylor, A. E. (1967). Bidirectional movement of water through the skin of a non-sweating animal. *J. Surgical Res.*, **7**, 323–328.

Negherbon, W. O. (1959). *Handbook of Toxicology* Vol. 3. Saunders—London.

Nelson, D. L. (1977). 'Pesticide safety as it relates to the manufacturing, warehousing and distribution of pesticides' in *Pesticide Management and Insecticide Resistance*. Editors: D. C. Watson and A. W. A. Brown. Academic Press—N.Y., San Francisco, and London.

Nelson, W., Kupferberg, H. and Halberg, F. (1971). Dose–response evaluations of a circadian rhythmic change in susceptibility of mice to ouabain. *Tox. Appl. Pharmacol.*, **18**, 335–339.

Neuhold, J. M. and Sigler, W. F. (1960). Effects of sodium fluoride on carp and rainbow trout. *Trans. Amer. Fish Soc.*, **89**, 358–370.

Newbold, C. (1975). Herbicides in aquatic systems. *Biol. Conserv.*, **7**, 97–118.

Niedner, R., Oettingen, V. von, and Meyer, F. (1974). Binding of warfarin on the serum proteins of mice and rats. *Naunym—Schmiedeberg's Arch. Pharmacol.*, **282**, R70.

Niessen, H., Tietz, H., Hecht, G. and Kimmerle, G. (1963). Uber Vorkommen von Sulfoniumverbindungen in Metasystox und Metasystox R und ihre physiologische Wirkung. *Arch. Toxicol.*, **20**, 44–60.

Nishiuchi, Y. and Yoshida, K. (1974). Effects of pesticides on tadpoles (in Japanese). *Noyaku Kensasho Hokoku*, **14**, 66–68.

Noakes, D. N. and Sanderson, D. M. (1969). A method for determining the dermal toxicity of pesticides. *Brit. J. industr. Med.*, **26**, 59–64.

Noel, P. R., Barnett, K. C., Davies, R. E., Jolly, D. W., Leahy, J. S., Mawdesley-Thomas, L. E., Schillam, K. W., Squires, P. F., Street, A. E., Tucker, W. C. and Worden, A. N. (1975). The toxicity of dimethylsulphoxide for the dog, pig, rat and rabbit. *Toxicology*, **3**, 143–169.

Noordhoek, J. and Rümke, C. L. (1969). Sex differences in the rate of drug metabolism in mice. *Arch. int. Pharmacodyn*, **182**, 401.

Nosal, M. and Hladka, A. (1968). Determination of the exposure to fenitrothion on the basis of the excretion of *p*-nitro-*m*-cresol by the urine of persons tested. *Arch. Gewerbepath. Gewerbehyg*, **25**, 28–38.

Nye, D. E. and Dorough, H. W. (1976). Fate of insecticides administered endotracheally to rats. *Bull. environ. Contam. Tox.*, **15**, 291–296.

Nyhan, W. L. (1961). Toxicity of drugs in the neo-natal period. *J. Pediat.*, **59**, 1–20.
O'Brien, R. D. and Dannelley, C. E. (1965). Penetration of insecticides through rat skin. *J. Agr. Food Chem.*, **13**, 245–247.
Occupational Health Notes (1963). Phosdrin contaminated clothing. *Public Health Rept.*, **78**, 260.
Okey, A. B. and Page, D. J. (1974). Acute toxicity of *o,p'*-DDT to mice. *Bull. environ. Contam. Toxicol.*, **11**, 359–363.
Oldendorf, W. H. (1974). Lipid solubility and drug penetration of the blood–brain barrier. *Proc. Soc. Exptl. Biol. Med.*, **147**, 813–816.
Onken, H. D. and Moyer, C. A. (1963). The water barrier in human epidermis: physical and chemical nature. *Arch. Derm.*, **87**, 584–590.
O'Reilly, W. J. (1972). Pharmacokinetics in drug metabolism and toxicology. *Canad. J. Pharm. Sci.*, **7**, 66–77.
Oreopoulos, D. G. and McEvoy, J. (1969). Diquat poisoning. *Post-grad. Med. J.*, **45**, 635.
Oser, B. L. (1971). 'Toxicology of pesticides to establish proof of safety' in *Pesticides in the Environment* Vol. 1. (Part 2). Editor: R. White-Stevens. Marcel Dekker Inc.—N.Y.
Ostrenga, J., Steinmetz, C. and Poulsen, B. (1971). Significance of vehicle composition: I. Relationship between topical vehicle composition, skin penetrability and clinical efficacy. *J. Pharm. Sci.*, **60**, 1175–1179.
Oudbier, A. J., Bloomer, A. W., Price, W. A. and Weich, R. L. (1974). Respiratory route of pesticide exposure as a potential health hazard. *Bull. Environ. Contam. Toxicol.*, **12**, 1–9.
Paget, G. E. and Barnes, J. M. (1964). 'Toxicity tests' in *Evaluation of Drug Activities: Pharmacometrics*. Editors: D. R. Laurence and A. L. Bacharach. Academic Press—London and N.Y.
Palmer, J. S. and Schlinke, J. C. (1973). Oral toxicity of tributyl phosphorotrithioite, a cotton defoliant to cattle and sheep. *J. Am. Vet. Med. Assoc.*, **163**, 1172–1174.
Pallotta, A. J., Kelly, M. G., Rall, D. P. and Ward, J. W. (1962). Toxicology of acetoxycycloheximide as a function of sex and body weight. *J. Pharmacol.*, **136**, 400–405.
Pan, H. P. and Fouts, J. R. (1978). Drug metabolism in birds. *Drug Metab. Revs.*, **7**, 1–253.
Pappenheimer, J. R. (1953). Passage of molecules through capillary walls. *Physiol. Revs.*, **33**, 387–423.
Parker, V. H., Barnes, J. M. and Denz, F. A. (1951). Some observations on the toxic properties of 3,5-dinitro-orthocresol. *Brit. J. industr. Med.*, **8**, 226–235.
Pekas, J. C. and Giles, J. L. (1974). Effect of dosing technique on absorption of carbaryl. *Fd Cosmet. Toxicol.*, **12**, 169.
Pellegrini, G. and Santi, R. (1972). Potentiation of toxicity of organophosphorus compounds containing carboxylic ester functions towards warm-blooded animals by some organophosphorus impurities. *J. Agr. Food Chem.*, **20**, 944–950.
Penniston, J. T., Beckett, L., Bentley, D. L. and Hansch, C. (1969). Passive permeation of organic compounds through biological tissue: A non-steady state theory. *Mol. Pharmacol.*, **5**, 333–341.
Peregrine, D. J. (1973). Toxic baits for the control of pest animals. *PANS*, **19**, 523–533.
Perlman, P. L. (1970). Transfer of animal pharmacology and toxicology data to man. *Drug Inf. Bull.*, **4**, 7–9.
Peters, R. A. (1963). *Biochemical Lesions and Lethal Synthesis*. Pergamon Press—Oxford, London, N.Y., and Paris.
Petrella, V. J., Fox, J. P. and Webb, R. E. (1975). Endrin metabolism in endrin-susceptible and resistant strains of pine mice. *Tox. Appl. Pharmacol.*, **34**, 283–291.
Pickering, C. E. and Pickering, R. G. (1971). Methods for the estimation of acetylcholinesterase activity in the plasma and brain of laboratory animals given carbamates or organophosphorus compounds. *Arch. Toxicol.*, **27**, 292–310.
Pickering, C. E. and Pickering, R. G. (1977). The interference of erythrocyte 'acetylcholinesterase' in the estimation of the blood cholinesterase activity of the chicken. *Tox. Appl. Pharmacol.*, **39**, 229–237.
Pickering, R. G. and Pickering, C. E. (1974). Methods for the estimation of acetylcholinesterase activity in the erythrocytes of laboratory animals given carbamates or organophosphorus compounds. *Arch. Toxicol.*, **31**, 197–216.
Pickering, W. R. (1965). The acute toxicity of chlorfenvinphos to sheep and cattle when applied dermally. *Vet. Rec.*, **77**, 1140–1144.
Pillmore, R. E. (1973). 'Toxicity of pyrethrum to fish and wildlife' in *Pyrethrum—The Natural Insecticide*. Editor: J. E. Casida. Academic Press—N.Y. and London.

146

Piotrowski, J. (1972). *The Application of Metabolic and Excretion Kinetics to Problems of Industrial Toxicology.* (U.S. Dept. of Health, Education and Welfare—Washington, D.C.).

Plackett, R. L. and Hewlett, P. S. (1948). Statistical aspects of the independent joint action of poisons, particularly insecticides. *Ann. Appl. Biol.*, **35**, 347–358.

Plackett, R. L. and Hewlett, P. S. (1952). Quantal response to mixtures of poisons. *J. Roy. Stat. Soc. (B)*, **14**, 141–163.

Plackett, R. L. and Hewlett, P. S. (1967). A comparison of two approaches to the construction models for quantal responses to mixtures of drugs. *Biometrics*, **23**, 27–44.

Pope, G. G. and Ward, P. (1972). The effects of small applications of an organophosphorus poison fenthion on the weaver bird (*Quelea quelea*). *Pestic. Sci.*, **3**, 197–205.

Potts, A. M. (1965). 'The effects of drugs upon the eye' in *Physiological Pharmacology* Vol. 2. Editors: W. S. Root and F. G. Hofman. Academic Press—N.Y. and London.

Prescott, L. F. (1972). 'Pharmacokinetic drug interactions—Mechanisms of toxicity'. *Proc. 14th Meeting European Society for the Study of Drug Toxicity* (Utrecht—Netherlands).

Prescott, L. F., Nimmo, W. S. and Heading, R. C. (1977). 'Drug absorption interactions' in *Drug Interactions*. Editor: D. G. Graham-Smith. (Macmillan Press Ltd.—London).

Princi, F. (1964). Criteria for the evaluation of chemical toxicity. *J. Air Pollut. Contr. Assoc.*, **14**, 154–157.

Pyle, N. J. (1940). Use of ferrets in laboratory work and research investigations. *Amer. J. Public Health*, **30**, 787–796.

Quinby, G. E. and Lemmon, A. B. (1958). Parathion residues as a cause of poisoning in crop workers. *J. Amer. Med. Assoc.*, **166**, 740–746.

Quinn, G. P., Axelrod, J. and Brodie, B. B. (1958). Species, strain and sex differences in metabolism of hexobarbitone, amidopyrine, antipyrine and aniline. *Biochem. Pharmacol.*, **1**, 152–159.

Quinones, M. A., Bogden, J. D., Louria, D. B. and Nakah, A. E. (1976). Depressed cholinesterase activities among farm workers in New Jersey. *Sci. Total Environ.*, **6**, 155–159.

Radeleff, R. D. (1970). *Veterinary Toxicology* 2nd Edition. Lea and Febriger—Philadelphia.

Radeleff, R. D. and Bushland, R. C. (1953). Benzene hexachloride poisoning of emaciated sheep. *Vet. Med.*, **48**, 53–58.

Radomski, J. L., Astolfi, E., Deichmann, W. B. and Rey, A. A. (1971). Blood levels of organochlorine pesticides in Argentina: Occupationally and non-occupationally exposed adults, children and newborn infants. *Tox. Appl. Pharmacol.*, **20**, 186–193.

Rainsford, K. D. (1978). Toxicity in the brain of organophosphate insecticides: Comparison of the toxicities of metabolites with parent compounds using an intracerebal injection method. *Pestic. Biochem. Physiol.*, **8**, 302–316.

Rall, D. P. (1969). Difficulties in extrapolating the results of toxicity studies in laboratory animals to man. *Environ. Res.*, **2**, 360–367.

Rall, D. P. (1971). 'Drug entry into brain and CSF' in *Handbook of Experimental Pharmacology*, **28**(2). Editors: B. B. Brodie and J. R. Gilette. Springer-Verlag—Berlin, Heidelberg, and N.Y.

Rall, D. P. and North, W. C. (1953). Consideration of dose–weight relationships. *Proc. Soc. exptl. Biol. Med.*, **83**, 825–827.

Ramachandran, B. V. (1966). Distribution of $DF^{32}P$ in mouse organs: (i) The effect of route of administration on incorporation and toxicity. *Biochem. Pharmacol.*, **15**, 169–175.

Ramakrishna, N. and Ramachandran, B. V. (1977). Potentiation of malathion toxicity by parathion. *Indian J. Biochem. Biophys.*, **14**, 53 only.

Reggiani, G. (1978). Medical problems raised by the TCDD contamination in Seseso, Italy. *Arch. Toxicol.*, **40**, 161–188.

Reichert, E. R., Klemmer, H. W. and Haley, T. J. (1978). A note on dermal poisoning from mevinphos and parathion. *Clin. Tox.*, **12**, 33–35.

Reiff, M. (1974). The laboratory screening of chemicals for toxicity to fish. *Proc. 16th Meeting European Society for the Study of Drug Toxicity*, (Carlsbad—CSSR).

Reiter, L., Talens, G. and Woolley, D. (1973). Acute and subacute parathion treatment: Effects on cholinesterase activities and learning in mice. *Tox. Appl. Pharmacol.*, **25**, 582–588.

Reiter, L., Talens, G. and Woolley, D. (1975). Parathion administration in the monkey: Time course of inhibition and recovery of blood cholinesterases and visual discrimination performance. *Tox. Appl. Pharmacol.*, **33**, 1–13.

Revzin, A. M. (1973a). Subtle changes in brain functions produced by single doses of mevinphos. *Report No. FAA-AM-75-3*, Federal Aviation Administration, Civil Aeromedical Institute, Oklahoma City, Oklahoma, U.S.A.

Revzin, A. M. (1973b). Transient blindness due to the combined effects of mevinphos and atropine. *Report No. FAA-AM-73-4*, Federal Aviation Administration, Civil Aeromedical Institute, Oklahoma City, Oklahoma, U.S.A.

Revzin, A. M. (1976a). Effects of mevinphos (PHOSDRIN) on unit discharge patterns in avian hippocampus. *Aviation, Space, Environ. Med.*, **47**, 608–611.

Revzin, A. M. (1976b). Effects of organophosphate pesticides and other drugs on subcortical mechanisms of visual integration. *Aviation, Space, Environ. Med.*, **47**, 627–629.

Rich, S. T. (1968). The Mongolian gerbil (*Meriones unguiculatus*) in research. *Lab. Anim. Care*, **18**, 235–243.

Rider, J. A., Moeller, H. C., Puletti, E. J. and Swader, J. I., (1969). Toxicity of parathion, systox, octamethyl pyrophosphoramide and methyl parathion in man. *Tox. Appl. Pharmacol.*, **14**, 603–611.

Riegelman, S. and Rowland, M. (1974). Effect of route of administration on drug disposition. *J. Pharmacokin. Biopharm.*, **1**, 419–434.

Riihimäki, V. and Pfäffli, P. (1978). Percutaneous absorption of solvent vapors in man. *Scand. J. Work Environ. Hlth.*, **4**, 73–85.

Ritschel, W. A., Siegel, E. G. and Ring, P. E. (1974). Biopharmaceutical factors influencing LD_{50}: Pt. 1 Viscosity. *Arzneim.—Forsch*, **24**, 907–910.

Ritter, C., Hughes, R., Snyder, G. and Weaver, L. (1970). Dichlorvos-containing dog collars and thiamylal anaesthesia. *Amer. J. Vet. Res.*, **31**, 2025–2027.

Roberts, M. S., Shorley, C. D., Arnold, R. and Anderson, R. A. (1974). The percutaneous absorption of phenolic compounds: I. Aqueous solutions of phenol in the rat. *Aust. J. Pharm. Sci.*, **NS3**, 81–91.

Robinson, C. P., Smith, P. W., Crane, C. R., McConnell, J. K., Allen, L. V. and Endecott, B. R. (1978). The protective effects of ethylestrenol against acute poisoning by organophosphorus cholinesterase inhibitors in rats. *Arch. int. Pharmacodyn.*, **231**, 168–176.

Robinson, F. R., Harper, D. T. and Kaplan, H. P. (1967). Comparison of strains of rats exposed to oxygen at various pressures. *Lab. Anim. Care*, **17**, 433–441.

Robinson, J., Richardson, A., Bush, B. and Elgar, K. E. (1966). A photoisomerization product of dieldrin. *Bull. environ. Contam. Toxicol.*, **1**, 127–132.

Rodnitzky, R. L. (1974). 'Neurological and behavioral aspects of occupational exposure to organophosphate pesticides' in *Behavioral Toxicology*. Editors: C. Xintaras, B. L. Johnson and I. de Groot. U.S. Dept. of Health, Education and Welfare, Public Health Service Center for Disease Control N.I.O.S.H.—Washington, D.C.

Rodnitzky, R. L., Levin, H. S. and Mick, D. L. (1975). Occupational exposure to organophosphate pesticides. *Arch. environ. Hlth.*, **30**, 98–103.

Rogers, P. A. M., Spillane, T. A., Fenlow, M. and Henaghan, T. (1973). Suspected paraquat poisoning in pigs and dogs. *Vet. Rec.*, **93**, 44–45.

Rose, M. S. (1975). The search for an effective treatment of paraquat poisoning. *Chem. Industr. (London)*, **10**, 413–415.

Rosen, J. D. and Sutherland, D. J. (1967). The nature and toxicity of the photoconversion products of aldrin. *Bull. environ. Contam. Toxicol.*, **2**, 1–9.

Rosen, J. D., Sutherland, D. J. and Lipton, G. R. (1966). The photochemical isomerization products of dieldrin and endrin and effects on toxicity. *Bull. environ. Contam. Toxicol.*, **1**, 133–140.

Rosenberg, P. and Coon, J. M. (1958). Increase of hexobarbital sleeping time by certain anticholinesterases. *Proc. Soc. Exptl. Biol. Med.*, **98**, 650–652.

Roszkowski, A. P. (1965). The pharmacological properties of norbormide, a selective rat toxicant. *J. Pharmacol. exptl. Ther.*, **149**, 288–299.

Roszkowski, A. P. (1967). Comparative toxicity of rodenticides. *Fedn. Proc.*, **26**, 1082–1088.

Rothman, S. (1943). The principles of percutaneous absorption. *J. Lab. Clin. Med.*, **28**, 1305–1321.

Rothman, S. (1955). The mechanism of percutaneous penetration and absorption. *J. Soc. Cosmet. Chemists*, **6**, 193–200.

Rothschild, Lord. (1961). *A Classification of Living Animals*. Longmans—London.

Rowland, M. (1972). Influence of route of administration on drug availability. *J. Pharm. Sci.*, **61**, 70–74.

148

Russell, R. W., Watson, R. H. J. and Frankenhauser, M. (1961). Effects of chronic reductions in brain cholinesterase activity on acquisition and estimation of a conditioned avoidance response. *Scand. J. Psychol.*, **2**, 21–29.

Sacher, G. A. and Trucco, E. (1962). The stochastic theory of mortality. *Ann. N.Y. Acad. Sci.*, **96**, 985–1007.

Sachsse, K. and Hess, R. (1972). Exposure of volunteers and animals in aerial application test of phosphamidon (DIMECRON 100) in India. *Proc. 14th Meeting European Society for the Study of Drug Toxicity* (Utrecht—Netherlands).

Sachsse, K., Ullmann, L., Voss, G. and Hess, R. (1973a). Measurement of inhalation toxicity of aerosols in laboratory animals. *Proceedings, 15th Meeting, European Society for the Study of Drug Toxicity* (Zurich—Switzerland).

Sachsse, K., Voss, G. and Hess, R. (1973b). Testing aerosols for inhalation toxicity in small laboratory animals. *Proceedings, 1st International Congress on Aerosols in Medicine* (Baden/Wien, Austria—September 1973).

Safarov, Y. B. and Aleskerov, S. A. (1972). Effect of pesticides in producing relapses in animals recovering from bacterial infections (in Russian). *Probl. Vet. Sanit.*, **43**, 213–218.

Sanderson, D. M. (1959). Glycerol formal as a solvent in toxicity testing. *J. Pharm. Pharmacol.*, **11**, 150–156.

Saunders, D. R., Paolino, R. M., Bousquet, W. F. and Miya, T. S. (1974). Age-related responsiveness of the rat to drugs affecting the CNS. *Proc. Soc. exptl Biol. Med.*, **147**, 593–595.

Scaife, J. F. and Campbell, D. H. (1958). Toxicity of a cholinesterase inhibitor to the hibernating hamster. *Nature*, **182**, 1739.

Schafer, E. W. (1972). The acute oral toxicity of 369 pesticidal, pharmaceutical and other chemicals to wild birds. *Tox. Appl. Pharmacol.*, **21**, 315–330.

Schafer, E. W. and Cunningham, D. J. (1972). An evaluation of 148 compounds as avian immobilizing agents. Special Scientific Report—*Wildlife No. 150*. (U.S. Dept. of Interior, Fish and Wildlife Service, Washington, D.C.).

Schafer, Jr., E. W., Bunton, R. B., Lockyer, N. F. and De Grazio, J. W. (1973). Comparative toxicity of seventeen pesticides to the Quelea, house sparrow and red-winged blackbird. *Tox. Appl. Pharmacol.*, **26**, 154–157.

Schanker, L. S. (1960). On the mechanism of absorption of drugs from the gastrointestinal tract. *J. Med. Pharm. Chem.*, **2**, 343–359.

Scheline, R. R. (1968). Drug metabolism by intestinal microorganisms. *J. Pharm. Sci.*, **57**, 2021–2037.

Scheuplein, R. J. (1965). Mechanism of percutaneous absorption. (i) Routes of penetration and the influence of solubility. *J. Invest. Derm.*, **45**, 334–346.

Scheuplein, R. J. (1967). Mechanism of percutaneous absorption. (ii) Transient diffusion and the relative importance of various routes of skin penetration. *J. Invest. Derm.*, **48**, 79–88.

Scheuplein, R. J. and Blank, I. H. (1971). Permeability of the skin. *Physiol. Rev.*, **51**, 302–747.

Scheuplein, R. and Ross, L. W. (1970). Effect of surfactants and solvents on the permeability of epidermis. *J. Soc. Cosmet. Chem.*, **21**, 853–873.

Scheuplein, R. J. and Ross, L. W. (1974). Mechanism of percutaneous absorption. (V) Percutaneous absorption of solvent deposited solids. *J. Invest. Derm.*, **62**, 353–360.

Scheving, L. E., Mayerbach, H. V. and Pauly, J. E. (1974). An overview of chronopharmacology. *J. Europ. Toxicol.*, **7**, 203–227.

Schlinke, J. C. and Palmer, J. S. (1972). Toxicity of two organophosphorus insecticides in stressed cattle. *J. Econ. Entomol.*, **65**, 64–66.

Schneiderman, M. A., Mantel, N. and Brown, C. C. (1975). From mouse to man—or how to get from the laboratory to Park Avenue and 59th Street. *Ann. N.Y. Acad. Sci.*, **246**, 237–248.

Schrader, G. (1961). Zur Kenntris neuer wenig toxischer Insektizide auf der Basis von Phosphorsäureestern. *Angew. Chem.*, **10**, 331–334.

Schroeder, C. R. (1967). Potential species new to laboratory investigation. *Fed. Proc.*, **26**, 1157–1161.

Secher-Hansen, E., Langgard, H. and Schou, J. (1967a). Studies on the subcutaneous absorption in mice I—a method for studying quantitatively the dynamics of subcutaneous absorption. *Acta pharmacol. Toxicol.*, **25**, 162–168.

Secher-Hansen, E., Langgard, H. and Schou, J. (1967b). Studies on the subcutaneous absorption in mice II—influence of toxicity on the dynamics of subcutaneous absorption. *Acta pharmacol. Toxicol.*, **25**, 290–298.

Selisko, O., Hentschel, G. and Ackermann, H. (1963). Uber die abhängigkeit der mittleren Tödlichen Dosis (LD$_{50}$) von exogenen Faktoren. *Arch. Int. Pharmacodyn. Therap.*, **45**, 51–69.

Sellassie, M. A. G. and Lester, F. (1971). Malathion poisoning. *Ethiop. Med. J.*, **9**, 205–206.

Serat, W. F. (1973). Calculation of a safe re-entry time into an orchard treated with a pesticide chemical which produces a measurable physiological response. *Arch. environ. Contam. Toxicol.*, **1**, 170–181.

Serat, W. F., Mengle, D. C., Anderson, H. P., Kahn, E. and Bailey, J. B. (1975). On the estimation of worker entry intervals into pesticide treated fields with and without the exposure of human subjects. *Bull. environ. Contam. Toxicol.*, **13**, 506–512.

Seume, F. W. and O'Brien, R. D. (1960a). Potentiation of the toxicity to insects and mice of phosphorothionates containing carboxyester and carboxyamide groups. *Tox. Appl. Pharmacol.*, **2**, 495–503.

Seume, F. W. and O'Brien, R. D. (1960b). Metabolism of malathion by rat tissue preparations and its modification by EPN. *J. Agr. Food Chem.*, **8**, 36–41.

Shaffer, C. B. and West, B. (1960). The acute and subacute toxicity of technical *o,o*-diethyl *s*-2-diethyl-aminoethyl phosphorothioate hydrogen oxalate (TETRAM). *Tox. Appl. Pharmacol.*, **2**, 1–13.

Shah, P. V. and Guthrie, F. E. (1977). 'Dermal absorption, distribution and the fate of six pesticides in the rabbit' in *Pesticide Management and Insecticide Resistance*. Editors: D. L. Watson and A. W. A. Brown. Academic Press—N.Y., San Francisco, and London.

Shakman, R. A. (1974). Nutritional influences on the toxicity of environmental pollutants. *Arch. environ. Hlth.*, **28**, 105–113.

Shanor, S. P., van Hees, G. R., Baart, N., Erdös, E. G. and Foldes, F. F. (1961). The influence of age and sex on human plasma and red cell cholinesterase. *Amer. J. Med. Sci.*, **242**, 357–361.

Sharp, C. W., Ottolenghi, A. and Posner, H. S. (1972). Correlation of paraquat toxicity with tissue concentrations and weight loss of the rat. *Tox. Appl. Pharmacol.*, **22**, 241–251.

Sherman, M., Ross, E. and Chang, M. T. Y. (1965). Acute and subacute toxicity of several insecticides to chicks. *Tox. Appl. Pharmacol.*, **7**, 606–608.

Shihab, K. (1976). Malathion poisoning among spraymen. *Bull. Endemic Dis.*, **17**, 69–74.

Sidorenko, G. I. and Pinigin, M. A. (1976). Concentration time relationship for various regimens of inhalation of organic compounds. *Environ. Health Perspect.*, **13**, 17–21.

Silverman, J. and Chavannes, J-M. (1977). Biological values of the European hamster (*Cricetus cricetus*). *Lab. Anim. Sci.*, **27**, 641–645.

Silverman, P. (1974). Behavioural toxicology. *New Scientist*, **61**, 255–257.

Simpson, G. R. and Penney, D. J. (1974). Pesticide poisonings in the Namoi and Macquarie valleys, 1973. *Med. J. Aust.*, **1**, 258–260.

Simpson, K. (1964). *Forensic Medicine*. Edward Arnold—London.

Simpson, R. E. and Simpson, G. R. (1969). Poisoning with monocrotophos, an organophosphorus pesticide. *Med. J. Austr.*, **2**, 1013–1016.

Sinow, J. and Wei, E. (1973). Ocular toxicity of paraquat. *Bull. environ. Contam. Toxicol.*, **9**, 163–168.

Skidmore, J. F. (1974). Factors affecting the toxicity of pollutants to fish. *Vet. Rec.*, **94**, 456–458.

Skinner, C. and Kilgore, W. (1978). Development of an animal model for prediction of agricultural field re-entry hazard. 17th Annual Meeting Society of Toxicology (San Francisco, March, 1978)—Abstract only.

Sladek, N. E., Chaplin, M. D. and Mannering, G. J. (1974). Sex-dependent differences in drug metabolism in the rat. IV. Effect of morphine administration. *Drug Metab. Disp.*, **2**, 293–300.

Smith, I. A. and Boyd, J. H. (1972). Another case of poisoning by alphachloralose. *Vet. Rec.*, **91**, 662.

Smith, L. L. and Rose, M. S. (1977). The toxicity of paraquat in mature and immature rats. *Proc. 16th Annual Meeting of the Society of Toxicology* (Toronto, Canada)—Abstract only.

Smith, L. L., Wright, A., Wyatt, I. and Rose, M. S. (1974). Effective treatment for paraquat poisoning in rats and its relevance to treatment of paraquat poisoning in man. *Br. Med. J.*, **4**, 569–571.

150

Smith, R. L. (1971). 'The role of the gut flora in the conversion of inactive compounds to active metabolites' in *Mechanisms of Toxicity*. Editor: W. N. Aldridge. Macmillan—London.

Smyth, D. H. (1964). 'Alimentary absorption of drugs: physiological considerations' in *Absorption and Distribution of Drugs*. Editor: T. B. Binns. E. and S. Livingstone Ltd.—Edinburgh and London.

Snow, D. H. (1973). The acute toxicity of dichlorvos in the dog: (ii) Pathology. *Austr. Vet. J.*, **49**, 120–125.

Snow, D. H. and Watson, A. D. J. (1973). The acute toxicity of dichlorvos in the dog: (i) clinical observations and clinical pathology. *Austr. Vet. J.*, **49**, 113–119.

Solomon, L. M., West, D. P., Fitzcoff, J. F. and Becker, A. M. (1977). Gamma benzene hexachloride in guinea pig brain after topical application. *J. Invest. Derm.*, **68**, 310–312.

Spector, W. S. (1956). *Handbook of Biological Data*. W. B. Saunders Co.—Philadelphia and London.

Spencer, E. Y. (1961). The dissimilar selective toxicity of two vinyl phosphorothionate isomers (Thionophosdrin). *Canad. J. Biochem. Physiol.*, **39**, 1790–1792.

Spratt, J. L. (1966). Computer program for probit analyses. *Tox. Appl. Pharmacol.*, **8**, 110–112.

Staiff, D. C., Irle, G. K. and Felsenstein, W. C. (1973). Screening of various adsorbents for protection against paraquat poisoning. *Bull. environ. Contam. Toxicol.*, **10**, 193–199.

Staiff, D. C., Comer, S. W., Armstrong, J. F. and Wolfe, H. R. (1975). Exposure to the herbicide paraquat. *Bull. environ. Contam. Toxicol.*, **14**, 334–340.

Starr, H. G. and Clifford, N. J. (1971). Absorption of pesticides in a chronic skin disease. *Arch. environ. Hlth.*, **22**, 398–400.

Starr, H. G. and Clifford, N. J. (1972). Acute lindane intoxication—a case study. *Arch. environ. Hlth.*, **25**, 384–375.

State of California, Dept. of Public Health Bureau of Occupational Health and Environmental Epidemiology. (1975). 'Occupational disease in California attributed to pesticides and other agricultural chemicals.'

Stave, U. (1964). Age dependent changes of metabolism. I. Studies of enzyme patterns of rabbit organs. *Biol. Neonat.*, **6**, 128–147.

Stavinhova, W. B., Weintraub, S. T. and Modak, A. T. (1974). Regional concentrations of choline and acetylcholine in the rat brain. *J. Neurochem.*, **23**, 885–886.

Steen, J. A., Hanneman, G. D., Nelson, P. L. and Folk, E. D. (1976). Acute toxicity of mevinphos to gerbils. *Tox. Appl. Pharmacol.*, **35**, 195–198.

Stevens, J. T., Stitzel, R. E. and McPhillips, J. J. (1972). Effects of anticholinesterase insecticides on hepatic microsomal metabolism. *J. Pharm. Pharmacol.*, **181**, 576–583.

Stevens, J. T., Farmer, J. D. and Dipasquale, L. C. (1978). The acute inhalation toxicity of technical capten and folpet. 17th Annual Meeting Society of Toxicology (San Francisco—March 1978) Abstract only.

Stevenson, D. E. and Carter, B. I. (1975). Pesticides and domestic animals. *Vet. Rec.*, **97**, 164–169.

Stockinger, H. E. (1953). Size of dose; its effect on distribution in the body. *Nucleonics*, **11**, 24–27.

Straub, K. D. (1974). A solid-state theory of oxidative phosphorylation. *J. theor. Biol.*, **44**, 191–206.

Stringer, J. G. (1968). Pesticide contamination of food and drugs during shipment. *FDA Papers*, **2**, 4–6.

Sun, Y-P. (1950). Toxicity Index—an improved method of comparing the relative toxicity of insecticides. *J. Econ. Entomol.*, **43**, 45–53.

Sussman, H. F., Cook, S. B. and Bloch, V. (1959). Human louse infestation: treatment with carbacide. *Arch. Derm.*, **100**, 82–83.

Swan, K. C. and White, N. G. (1942). Corneal permeability: (i) factors affecting penetration of drugs into the cornea. *Amer. J. Ophthalmol.*, **25**, 1043–1058.

Swoap, O. F. (1955). A collaborative study on the use of mice in acute toxicity testing. *J. Pharm. Sci.*, **44**, 11–16.

Szakall, A. (1951). Hautphysiologische Forschung und Gesunderhaltung der Haut. *Fette und Seifen.*, **53**, 399–405.

Szot, R. J. and Murphy, S. D. (1971). Relationships between cyclic variations in adrenocortical secretory activity in rats and the adrenocortical response to toxic chemical stress. *Environ. Res.*, **4**, 530–538.

Takano, Y. (1972). On the clinical cases of pesticide intoxication which were studied over five years beginning in 1967 (in Japanese). *Nippon Noson Igakkai Zasshi.*, **21**, 240–241.

Talanov, G. A. and Leshchev, V. V. (1972). Influence of formulation on the toxicity of BHC for warm blooded animals (in Russian). *Probl. Veter. Sanit.*, **41**, 216–223.

Tammes, P. M. L., Loosjes, F. E. and Wijnen, R. (1967). Time–response experiments with anticoagulants on rats. *Acta Physiol. Pharmacol. Neerl.*, **14**, 423–433.

Tanaka, K-I. (1971). Toxicity of dimethylformamide to the young female rat. *Int. Arch. Arbeitsmed.*, **28**, 95–105.

Tanner, J. M. (1949). Fallacy of per-weight and per-surface area standards and their relation to spurious correlation. *J. Appl. Physiol.*, **2**, 1–15.

Taylor, D. (1978). Dieldrin—poison threat that won't go away. *British Farmer and Stockbreeder* (19 August), 22.

Taylor, G. J. and Harris, W. S. (1970). Cardiac toxicity of aerosol propellants. *J. Am. Med. Assoc.*, **214**, 81–85.

Taylor, W., Guirgis, H. A. and Stewart, W. K. (1969). Investigation of population exposed to organomercurial seed dressings. *Arch. environ. Hlth.*, **19**, 505–509.

Tenney, S. M. and Remmers, J. E. (1963). Comparative quantitative morphology of the mammalian lung: Diffusing area. *Nature*, **197**, 54–56.

Thompson, W. R. (1947). Use of moving averages and interpolation to estimate median effective dose. *Bacteriol Rev.*, **11**, 115–145.

Thompson, W. R. and Weil, C. S. (1952). On the construction of tables for moving average interpolation. *Biometrics*, **8**, 51–54.

Thonney, M. L., Touchberry, R. W., Goodrich, R. D. and Meiske, J. C. (1974). Re-evaluation of metabolic body weight. *J. Anim. Sci.*, **39**, 1002.

Thorpe, E., Wilson, A. B., Dix, K. M. and Blair, D. (1972). Teratological studies with dichlorvos vapour in rabbits and rats. *Arch. Toxicol.*, **30**, 29–38.

Tobin, J. S. (1970). Carbofuran: A new carbamate insecticide. *J. Occup. Med.*, **12**, 16–19.

Tregear, R. T. (1962). The structures which limit the penetrability of the skin. *J. Soc. Cosmet. Chem.*, **13**, 145–151.

Tregear, R. T. (1964). 'The permeability of skin to molecules of widely-differing properties' in *Progress in the Biological Science in Relation to Dermatology*. Editors: A. Rook and R. H. Champion. Cambridge University Press—Cambridge.

Tregear, R. T. (1966a). *Physical Function of Skin*. Academic Press—London and N.Y.

Tregear, R. T. (1966b). The permeability of skin to albumin, dextrans and polyvinyl pyrrolidone. *J. Invest. Derm.*, **46**, 24–27.

Treon, J. F., Cleveland, F. P. and Cappel, J. (1955). Toxicity of endrin for laboratory animals. *J. Agr. Fd Chem.*, **3**, 842–848.

Triggs, E. J. and Nation, R. L. (1975). Pharmacokinetics in the aged: A review. *J. Pharmacokin. Biopharmaceut.*, **3**, 387–418.

Trinh-Van-Bao, Szabo, I., Ruzicska, P. and Czeizel, A. (1974). Chromosome observations in patients suffering acute organic phosphate insecticide intoxication. *Humangenetik*, **24**, 33–57.

Triolo, A. J. and Coon, J. M. (1963). Effects of aldrin and chlordane on the toxicity of organophosphates and hexobarbital sleeping time in mice. *Federation Proc.*, **22**, 189.

Truhaut, R., Gak, J-C. and Graillot, C. (1974). Recherches sur las modalites et les mechanismes d'action toxique des insecticides organochlores: I. Estude comparative des effets de toxicite aiguë chez le hamster et chez le rat. *J. Europ. Toxicol.*, **7**, 159–166.

Tucker, R. K. and Crabtree, D. G. (1970). *Handbook of Toxicity of Pesticides to Wildlife*. Bureau of Sport Fisheries and Wildlife—Resource Publication No. 84.

Tucker, R. K. and Haegele, M. A. (1971). Comparative acute oral toxicity of pesticides to six species of birds. *Tox. Appl. Pharmacol.*, **20**, 57.

Turtle, E. E. and Taylor, A. (1955). Chemicals against rodents and other animal pests. *Rep. Progr. Appl. Chem.*, **40**, 680–687.

Uchida, A., Ishige, T., Saito, M. and Oikawa, K. (1972). Results of the status of acute pesticide intoxications (in Japanese). *Nippon Noson Igakkai Zasshi*, **21**, 234–235.

Udall, N D. (1973). The toxicity of the molluscicides metaldehyde and methiocarb to dogs. *Vet. Rec.*, **93**, 420–422.

Ueteke, S., Yamada, K., Seta, K., Shirojura, T., Shigatani, R., Ogura, H., Satane, B. and Toyoda, O. (1972). A case of gramoxone intoxication (in Japanese). *Nippon Naika Gakkai Zasshi*, **61**, 1435–1436.

152

Umetsu, N., Grose, F. H., Allahyari, R., Sameer, A. and Fukuto, T. R. (1977). Effect of impurities on the mammalian toxicity of technical malathion and acephate. *J. Agric. Food Chem.*, **25**, 946–953.

Usinger, W. (1957). Respiratorischer Stoffwechsel und Körpertemperatur der weissen Mans in thermoindifferenter Umgebung. *Pflügers Archiv.*, **264**, 520–535.

Vaccarezza, J. R. and Peltz, L. (1960). Effect of ACTH on blood cholinesterase activity in normal subjects and respiratory-allergy patients. *Presse Med.*, **68**, 723–724.

Vaccarezza, J. R. and Willson, J. A. (1964a). The effect of ACTH on cholinesterase activity in plasma, whole blood and blood cells of rats. *Experientia*, **20**, 23.

Vaccarezza, J. R. and Willson, J. A. (1964b). The relationship between corticosterone administration and cholinesterase activity in rats. *Experientia*, **20**, 425.

Vaccarezza, J. R. and Willson, J. A. (1965). Blood cholinesterase in adrenalectomized rats. *Experientia*, **21**, 205.

Vandekar, M. (1958). The toxic properties of demeton-methyl (Metasystox) and some related compounds. *Brit. J. industr. Med.*, **15**, 158–167.

Vandekar, M. and Heath, D. F. (1957). The reactivation of cholinesterase after inhibition *in vivo* by some dimethyl phosphate esters. *Biochem. J.*, **67**, 202–208.

Vandekar, M. and Komanov, I. (1963). Study of dermal toxicity of organophosphorus compounds: (i) Parathion toxicity in relation to the skin surface and the technique of application (in Hungarian). *Arch. Hig. Rada*, **14**, 7–12.

Vandekar, M., Komanov, I. and Kobrehel, D. (1963). Study of dermal toxicity of organophosphorus compounds: (ii) Effect of the size of the contaminated skin area and the concentration of the poison in the penetration rate of paraoxon through the skin (in Hungarian). *Arch. Hig. Rada*, **14**, 13–18.

Vandekar, M., Reiner, E., Svetlicic, B. and Fajdetic, T. (1965). Value of ED_{50} testing in assessing hazards of acute poisoning by carbamates and organophosphates. *Brit. J. industr. Med.*, **22**, 317–320.

Vandekar, M., Plestina, R. and Wilhelm, K. (1971). Toxicity of carbamates for mammals. *Bull. Wld. Hlth. Org.*, **44**, 241–249.

Van Dijk, A., Maes, R. A. A., Drost, R. H., Douze, J. M. C. and van Heyst, A. N. P. (1975). Paraquat poisoning in man. *Arch. Toxicol.*, **34**, 129–136.

Van Gelder, G. A. (1975). 'Behavioral Toxicologic Studies of Dieldrin, DDT and Ruelene in Sheep', in *Behavioral Toxicology*. Plenum Press—N.Y. and London.

Van Harken, D. R. and Hottendorf, G. H. (1978). Comparative absorption following the administration of a drug to rats by oral gavage and incorporation in the diet. *Tox. Appl. Pharmacol.*, **43**, 407–410.

Veldstra, H. (1956). Synergism and potentiation with special reference to the combination of structural analogues. *Pharmacol. Rev.*, **8**, 339–389.

Venezky, D. L. (1971). A word of caution about use of dimethyl sulfoxide as solvent in analytical procedures. *Anal. Chem.*, **43**, 971.

Verschoyle, R. D. and Barnes, J. M. (1972). Toxicity of natural and synthetic pyrethrins to rats. *Pestic. Biochem. Physiol.*, **2**, 308–311.

Verschuuren, H. G., Kroes, R. and van Esch, G. J. (1973). Toxicity studies on tetrasul: (1) Acute, long-term and reproduction studies. *Toxicology*, **1**, 63–78.

Vessell, E. S. (1968). Genetic and environmental factors affecting hexobarbital metabolism in mice. *Ann. N.Y. Acad. Sci.*, **151**, 900–912.

Vessell, E. S. (1969). 'Recent progress in pharmacogenetics' in *Advances in Pharmacology and Chemotherapy* Vol. 7. Editors: S. Garattini, A. Goldin, F. Hawking and I. J. Kopin. Academic Press—N.Y. and London.

Vettorazzi, G. and Miles-Vettorazzi, P. (1975). Safety evaluation of chemicals in food: Toxicological data profiles for pesticides. (i) Carbamate and organophosphorus insecticides used in agriculture and public health. *Wld. Hlth. Orgn. Progress in Standardisation No. 3.*

Von Bertalanffy, L. (1951). Metabolic types and growth. *Amer. Naturalist*, **85**, 111–117.

Waitt, A. W. (1975). Pesticide legislation and industry. *Pestic. Sci.*, **6**, 199–208.

Walker, A. I. T. and Stevenson, D. E. (1968). Studies on the safety of plastic dog collars containing dichlorvos. *Vet. Rec.*, 23 November, 538–541.

Walker, A. I. T., Blair, D., Stevenson, D. E. and Chambers, P. L. (1972). An inhalational toxicity study with dichlorvos. *Arch. Toxicol.*, **30**, 1–8.

Walker, C. R. (1964). Dichlobenil as a herbicide in fish habitats. *Weeds*, **12**, 267–269.

Walsh, G. M. and Fink, G. B. (1972). Comparative toxicity and distribution of endrin and dieldrin after intravenous administration in mice. *Tox. Appl. Pharmacol.*, **23**, 408–416.

Ward, P. (1973). A new strategy for the control of damage by Queleas. *PANS*, **19**, 97–106.

Ware, G. W., Morgan, D. P., Estensen, B. J., Cahill, W. P. and Whitacre, D. M. (1973). Establishment of re-entry on human data: (I) Ethyl and methyl parathion. *Arch. environ. Contam. Toxicol.*, **1**, 48.

Ware, G. W., Morgan, D. P., Estesen, B. J. and Cahill, W. P. (1974). Establishment of re-entry intervals for organophosphate-treated cotton fields based on human data: (II) Azodrin, ethyl and methyl parathion. *Arch. environ. Contam. Toxicol.*, **2**, 117–129.

Wassermann, M., Wassermann, D., Gershon, Z. and Zeccermayer, L. (1969). Effects of organochlorine insecticides on body defence system. *Ann. N.Y. Acad. Sci.*, **160**, 393–401.

Watson, M., Benson, W. W. and Gabica, J. (1971). Accidental organophosphate poisoning in cattle. *Arch. Environ. Hlth.*, **22**, 582–583.

Waud, D. R. (1972). On biological assays involving quantal responses. *J. Pharm. exptl. Ther.*, **183**, 577–607.

Waud, D. R. (1975). 'Analysis of dose–response curves' in *Methods in Pharmacology* Vol. 3. Editors: E. E. Daniel and D. M. Paton. Plenum Press—N.Y. and London.

Way, J. M. (1969). Toxicity and hazards to man, domestic animals and wildlife from some commonly used auxin herbicides. *Res. Rev.*, **26**, 37–62.

Weaver, L. S. and Kerley, T. L. (1962). Strain difference in response to mice to *d*-amphetamine. *J. Pharm. exptl. Ther.*, **135**, 240–245.

Webb, R. E. and Horsfall, Jr. F. (1967). Endrin resistance in the pine mouse. *Science*, **156**, 1762.

Webb, R. E., Hartgrove, R. W., Randolph, W. L., Petrella, V. J. and Horsfall, Jr. F. (1973). Toxicity studies in endrin—susceptible and resistant strains of pine mice. *Tox. Appl. Pharmacol.*, **25**, 42–47.

Weber, T. and Berencsi, G. (1972). Data on safety gloves protection against pesticides (in German). *Int. Arch. Arbeitsmed.*, **30**, 23–30.

Weeks, D. E. (1967). Endrin food poisoning. *Bull. Wld. Hlth. Org.*, **37**, 499–512.

Weeks, M. H., Lawson, M. A., Angerhofer, R. A., Davenport, C. D. and Pennington, N. E. (1977). Preliminary assessment of the acute toxicity of malathion in animals. *Arch. Environ. Contam. Toxicol.*, **6**, 23–31.

Weidenbach, J. (1969). Vergiftung mit paraquat. *Deut. Med. Wochenschr.*, **94**, 545–547.

Weil, C. S. (1952). Tables for convenient calculation of median-effective dose (LD_{50} or ED_{50}) and instructions in their use. *Biometrics*, **8**, 249–263.

Weil, C. S. (1972a). Statistics vs safety factors and scientific judgement in the evaluation of safety for man. *Tox. Appl. Pharmacol.*, **21**, 454–463.

Weil, C. S. (1972b). Guidelines for experiments to predict the degree of safety of a material for man. *Tox. Appl. Pharmacol.*, **21**, 194–199.

Weil, C. S. (1975). Toxicology experimental design and conduct as measured by inter-laboratory collaborative studies. *J.A.O.A.C.*, **58**, 683–688.

Weil, C. S. and Wright, G. J. (1967). Intra- and interlaboratory comparative evaluation of single oral test. *Tox. Appl. Pharmacol.*, **11**, 378–388.

Weil, C. S., Carpenter, C. P. and Smyth, Jr., H. F. (1953). Specifications for calculating the median effective dose. *Am. industr. Hyg. Assoc. Quart.*, **14**, 200–206.

Weil, C. S., Carpenter, G. P., West, J. S. and Smyth, Jr., H. F. (1966). Reproducibility of single oral dose toxicity testing. *Amer. industr. Hyg. Assoc. J.*, **27**, 483–487.

Weil, C. S., Condra, N. I. and Carpenter, C. P. (1971). Correlation of 4-hour vs 24-hour contact skin penetration in the rat and rabbit and use of the former for predictions of relative hazard of pesticide formulations. *Tox. Appl. Pharmacol.*, **18**, 734–742.

Weinig, E. and Walz, W. (1971). Distribution of thallium in kidney and liver in lethal poisoning (in German). *Arch. Toxicol.*, **27**, 217–225.

Weinstock, M. and Shoham, S. (1974). Seasonal variation in sensitivity of guinea pig tissues to agonists. *Nature*, **251**, 427–428.

Weiss, L. R. and Orzel, R. A. (1967). Some comparative toxicological and pharmacologic effects of DMSO as a pesticide solvent. *Tox. Appl. Pharmacol.*, **11**, 546–557.

Wepierre, J. (1971). L'absorption percutanee. *Prod. Probl. Pharm.*, **26**, 312–327.

Wester, R. C. and Maibach, H. I. (1975). Percutaneous absorption in the Rhesus monkey compared to man. *Tox. Appl. Pharmacol.*, **32**, 394–398.

154

Westerfield, W. W. (1956). Biological response curves. *Science (Washington)*, **123**, 1017–1019.

White, I. N. H., Verschoyle, R. D., Moradian, M. H. and Barnes, J. M. (1976). The relationship between brain levels of cismethrin and bioresmethrin in female rats and neurotoxic effects. *Pestic. Biochem. Physiol.*, **6**, 491–500.

Whitehouse, L. W. and Ecobichon, D. J. (1975). Paraoxon formation and hydrolysis by mammalian liver. *Pestic. Biochem. Physiol.*, **5**, 314–322.

Whitton, J. T. and Everall, J. D. (1973). The thickness of the epidermis. *Br. J. Dermatol.*, **89**, 467–476.

W.H.O. Technical Report Series No. 513, (1973). *Safe Use of Pesticides*. 20th Report of the W.H.O. Expert Committee on Insecticides.

Wiberg, G. S. and Grice, H. C. (1965). Effect of prolonged individual caging on toxicity parameters in rats. *Fd Cosmet. Toxicol.*, **3**, 597–603.

Wiese, I. H., Basson, N. C. J., Basson, P. A., Naude, T. W. and Maartens, B. P. (1973). The toxicology and pathology of dieldrin and photodieldrin poisoning in two antelope species. *Onderstepoort J. Vet. Res.*, **40**, 31–40.

Wilkinson, G. T. (1973). Dieldrin poisoning in the cat. *Vet. Rec.*, **92**, 510.

Wilks, L. P. (1971). The meaning of LD_{50}. *Pesticides Annual*—December 1971.

Wills, J. H. (1968). 'Pharmacology' in *The Golden Hamster—its Biology and Use in Medical Research*. Editors: R. A. Hoffman, P. F. Robinson and H. Magalhaes. Iowa State Univ. Press—Ames, Iowa.

Wills, J. H., James, E. and Coulston, F. (1968). Effects of oral doses of carbaryl in man. *Clin. Toxicol.*, **1**, 265–271.

Wilson, E. B. and Worcester, J. (1943a). Bioassay on a general curve. *Proc. Nat. Acad. Sci.*, **29**, 150–154.

Wilson, E. B. and Worcester, J. (1943b). The determination of LD_{50} and its sampling error in bioassay. *Proc. Nat. Acad. Sci.*, **29**, Pt. 1. 79–85; Pt. 2. 114–120; Pt. 3. 257–262.

Wilson, F. A. and Dietschy, J. M. (1974). The intestinal unstirred layer—its surface area and effect on active transport kinetics. *Biochem. Biophys. Acta*, **363**, 112–126.

Wilson, J. (1966). *Thinking with Concepts*. Cambridge University Press.

Winfree, A. T. (1975). Unclocklike behaviour of biological clocks. *Nature*, **253**, 315–319.

Winne, D. (1970). Formal kinetics of water and solute absorption with regard to intestinal blood flow. *J. theor. Biol.*, **27**, 1–18.

Winne, D. (1978). Dependence of intestinal absorption *in vivo* in the unstirred layer. *Nauyn-Schmiedeberg's Arch. Pharmacol.*, **304**, 175–181.

Witschi, H. P. and Kacew, S. (1974). Studies on the pathological biochemistry of lung parenchyma in acute paraquat poisoning. *Med. Biol.*, **52**, 104–110.

Wohlrab, W., Marculescu, J. and Schneider, I. (1967). Zur Frage der Identität der epidermalen Barriere und der Intermediärzone menselicher Haut. *Archiv. Klin. exptl Derm.*, **230**, 432–436.

Wolfe, H. R. (1972a). Protection of workers from exposure to pesticides. *Pest. Control*, **40**, 17–42.

Wolfe, H. R. (1972b). 'Protection of individuals who mix or apply pesticides in the field'. *Proc. Nat. Conf. on Protective Clothing and Safety Equipment for Pesticide Workers* (Federal Working Group on Pest Management), Rockville, Md, U.S.A.

Wolfe, H. R., Durham, W. F. and Batchelor, G. S. (1961). Health hazards of some dinitro compounds. *Arch. environ. Hlth.*, **3**, 104–111.

Wolfe, H. R., Armstrong, J. F. and Durham, W. F. (1966). Pesticide exposure from concentrate spraying. *Arch. environ. Hlth.*, **13**, 340–344.

Wolfe, H. R., Durham, W. F. and Armstrong, J. F. (1967). Exposure of workers to pesticides. *Arch. environ. Hlth.*, **14**, 622–635.

Wolter, K., Schaefer, H., Fromming, K-H. and Stuttgen, G. (1972). Particle size and permeation. *Amer. Cosmet. Perf.*, **87**, 45–47.

Wood, S. G., Upshall, D. G. and Bridges, J. W. (1978). The absorption of aliphatic carbamates from the rat colon. *J. Pharm. Pharmac.*, **30**, 638–641.

Wood, W. W., Brown, H. W., Watson, M. (1971). Implication of organophosphate pesticide poisoning in the plane crash of a duster pilot. *Aerosp. Med.*, **42**, 111–113.

Worcester, J. and Wilson, E. B. (1943). A table determining LD_{50} or the 50% end-point. *Proc. Nat. Acad. Sci.*, **29**, 207–212.

Worden, A. N. (1969). Toxicity of telodrin. *Tox. Appl. Pharmacol.*, **14**, 556–573.

Worden, A. N. and Harper, K. H. (1964). Oral toxicity as influenced by method of administration. *Proc. 4th Symposium Europ. Soc. Study of Drug Toxicity*, (Cambridge—England).

World Health Organization (1972). *Modern Trends in the Prevention of Pesticide Intoxication.* W.H.O. Regional Office for Europe—Copenhagen.

Worthley, E. G. and Schott, C. D. (1966). Pharmacotoxic evaluation of nine vehicles administered intraperitoneally to mice. *Lloydia*, **29**, 123–129.

Wurster, D. E. and Dempski, R. E. (1961). Permeability of excised human keratin to lipid-soluble substances. *J. Pharm. Sci.*, **50**, 588–591.

Wysocka-Paruszewska, B., Osicka-Koprowska, A., Brzezinski, J. and Gradowska-Olszewska, I. (1979). Studies on the combined action in evaluation of pesticide toxicity. *21st Congress of the European Society of Toxicology* (Dresden, DDR). Proceedings to be published.

Yeary, R. A. (1967). Drug toxicity in newborn animals. *Appl. Therap.*, **9**, 918–921.

Yeary, R. A., Benish, R. A. and Finkelstein, M. (1966). Acute toxicity of drugs in newborn animals. *J. Pediat.*, **69**, 663–667.

Yegiazarov, G. M. (1971). Pesticides deployed by the U.S. Army in Vietnam (in Russian). *Voenno Med. Zh.*, **12**, 76–78.

Youden, W. J. (1963). Ranking laboratories by round robin tests. *Mater. Res. Std.*, **3**, 9–13.

Young, R., Jr., Johnson, L. G. and Brown, L. J. (1970). Pentobarbital sodium in the sleeping time of dogs wearing placebo or dichlorvos-containing flea control collars. *Vet. Med. (Small Animal Clinic)*, **65**, 609.

Zaeva, G. N., Timofievskaya, L. A., Stasenkova, K. P. and Bazarova, L. A. (1968). Utilization of time–effect curves in toxicology experiments (in Russian). *Toksikol. Novykh. Promyshbennykh Khimichesk. Veshchestr.*, Pages 5–9.

Zaroslinski, J. F., Browne, R. J. and Possley, L. H. (1971). Propylene glycol as a drug solvent in pharmacologic studies. *Tox. Appl. Pharmacol.*, **19**, 573–578.

Zeuthen, E. (1953). Oxygen uptake and body size in organisms. *Quart. Rev. Biol.*, **28**, 1–11.

Zimmermann, A. Matschiner, J. T. (1974). Biochemical basis of hereditary resistance to warfarin in the rat. *Biochem. Pharmacol.*, **23**, 1033–1040.

Index

Absorption, active transport and, 91
  alimentary, 89–94, 106
  buccal, 88–89
  convective, 91
  dermal, 94–106
  facilitated, 91–93
  gastro-intestinal tract and, 89–94, 106
  lymphatic system and, 91
  metabolism and, 109, 111–112
  parenteral administration and,
    111–113
  passive, 90
  percutaneous, 94–106
  pinocytosis and, 91
  respiratory tract and, 107–111
  through eyes, 106–107
  through skin, 94–106
Active transport, absorption from
    gastro-intestinal tract, 91
  skin penetration and, 97
Acute, definition of, 1, 107–108
Acute toxicity, bird embryos used in, 5
  classification of chemicals by, 10, 23
  data bank for, 5
  inaminate techniques for, 5, 120
  objectives of tests for, 4–5
  organ culture and, 5
  routes of exposure and, 88–113
  tissue culture used in, 5
Additive effects, 25–28, 74–80
Aerosols, inhalation of, 109
Age, epidermal thickness and, 99
  response related to, 51–56
  skin penetrability and, 56
Alimentary tract, see Gastro-intestinal
    tract
Allometric relationships, 46–51
Ambient conditions, influence on
    response, 63–67
Amphibians, toxicity of chemicals to, 45
Animals, availability of species for
    predictive tests, 34–45
  general, 33–63
  numbers of needed for predictive
    tests, 18–25

Antagonistic effect, definition of, 27–74
  interpretation of, 25
Aspiration, of vapours and fluids into
    respiratory tract, 107
Avian toxicity, see Birds
Avicides, assessment of, 41, 65, 82

Baits (toxic), dangers of, 82, 86
  pesticides used in, 82, 118
Behavioural effects, memory and
    concentration, 14, 87, 117
Bias, physiological, 45
Bioavailability, general, 73
  safety related to, 3
Birds, as pests, 82
  predictive toxicity tests using, 41–43,
    55
  species differences in response to
    toxicants, 41–43
Blood–brain barrier, penetration of by
    toxicants, 37, 56, 62, 68
Body, dose and effect
    relationship, 46–51
  surface area, 47, 70
Bodyweight, determining principle of, 49
  importance of in acute toxicity, 47, 68,
    116
  metabolic, 48
Buccal cavity, absorption in 88–89

Calculations, computerized, 22
  graphical methods in, 19–21
  logistic function in, 21
  'moving averages' in, 19
  Probits, use of, 19–21
  Ridits, use of, 22
  stochastic methods in, 22
Categorization of pesticides, by acute
    toxicity, 10, 23, 93, 104, 115
Children, fatalities due to pesticides, 7–8
Cholinesterases, age differences and, 52
  population differences, 52, 58
  sex differences and, 58
  stress and, 61

Clothing, contaminated, 84 87
  protective, limitations of, 85, 117
Coalitive effect, definition of, 27
Computer, as data bank, 120
  use of to predict acute toxicity, 5, 10
Concentration (mental), effects of
  pesticides on, 14, 87, 117
Concentration (of toxicant), effects on
  acute toxicity, 74, 92
  lethal (LC), 71
  relationship to time of exposure,
    70–71
Confidence limits, definition of, 22
Containers, contaminated, disposal of,
  84
  misuse of, 87
  unlabelled, cause of accidents 83
  unsuitable, cause of accidents, 87
Crops, losses due to pests, 6
Cruelty to Animals Act, 1876, Home
  Office enquiry into 'LD$_{50}$ test', 4

Death, definition of, 3
Dermal, *see* Skin
Diffusion, Fick's Law of, 97–98
  in skin penetration, 97–99
Dimethyl sulphoxide, solvent for acute
  toxicity tests, 75–77
Dioxins 9, 114, 118–119
Distribution, of toxicants in the body,
  61, 68, 70, 112
Dosage, definition of, 68
  units of, 68
Dose, definition of, 68
  response curves, 19–21
  selection of, 24
  sublethal, 79–80

Ecological effects 33, 34
Effect dose (ED) definition of, 17
  median (MED) 17
Effects, adaptive, 2
  additive, 25
  antagonistic, 27
  beneficial, 2
  coalitive, 27
  harmful, 2
  interactive, 25–28
  physiological, 2
  sub-lethal, 12, 14, 87, 117
Equipment, protective, 85, 117
Ethnic, considerations in relation to
  pesticide intoxication, 7–9, 117

Explosions, pesticide intoxication
  associated with, 9
Exposure, adventitious, 14, 34, 84–88,
  94, 115
  containers and, 10, 83, 87
  contaminated food and, 9, 87
  definition of acute, 1
  deliberate, 12, 81–84, 94
  diagnostic, 84, 94
  environmental, 70
  hazards of, 81–88
  inhalation, 70, 107–111
  monitoring, 12
  multiple, 1, 79–80, 90
  oral, 88–94
  parenteral, 88, 111–113, 115
  peroral, 88–94
  percutaneous, 94–106
  perocular, 106–107
  predictive tests and, 70, 88, 115
  routes of, 88–113
  therapeutic, 83
Eyes, absorption of toxicants through,
  106–107

Fiducial limits definition of, 22
Fires, pesticide intoxication associated
  with, 9, 115
Fish, pesticides used to kill, 43
  predictive toxicity tests using, 43–45,
    56
  toxicity of pesticides to, 43–45
Food, intoxication due to contaminated,
  9, 87
Food-chain effect, in acute toxicity, 86
Formulation, adsorbants in, 73
  complex formation to achieve, 73
  influence on acute toxicity, 71–78,
    118–119
  of toxicants for predictive tests, 75
  solubilization to achieve, 73

Gastro-intestinal tract, absorption of
  toxicants in, 89–94
  species differences, 92
Genetic effects, *see* Pharmacogenetics
Grain, intoxication due to pesticide
  contaminated, 87

Hazard, assessment, 115
  definition of, 1, 11
  exposure and, 81–88, 115, 120
Humidity, effects on acute toxicity, 66

Impurities, toxic in products, 114, 119
Inhalation, as route of exposure,
    107–111
Interactive effects, data due to, 25–28
    in percutaneous toxicity, 98
Isoboles, definition of, 27

Lethal concentration (LC), definition of,
    24
Lethal dose (LD), definition of, 17
    estimation of values, 17–28
    median (MLD), 17
    the 'LD$_{50}$ test', 4, 17, 120
'Lethal redistribution', importance of, 16
'Lethal synthesis', occurrence of, 16, 31
Life, definition of, 3
Limits, confidence, 22
    fiducial, 22

Man, sensitivity in relation to other
    species, 48
    value of animal models for predicting
    toxic effects in, 48
Manslaughter, by use of pesticides, 81
'Metabolic body weight', definition of,
    48
'Metabolic rate, basal, 51
Metabolism, of toxicants, 68–69
Mixtures, of toxicants, 25–28, 79–80
Models, use of biomathematical in the
    prediction of acute toxicity, 11, 17
Molecular weight, related to acute
    toxicity, 10
Mouth, absorption in, 88–89
Murder, by use of pesticides, 81

Neonates, sensitivity to acute
    intoxication, 52–54
Nutritional effects 58, 61–62

'Ontogenetic recapitulation', 48, 63

Paracelsus, ideas in toxicity, 2
Parenteral exposure, in experimental
    toxicology, 50
Particles, absorption of, 91–92
Particle size, importance in inhalation,
    109–110
Partition coefficient, absorption and, 89,
    97–98, 101–104
Percutaneous absorption, see Skin
Pesticides, classification by hazard, 32
    definition of, 2
    disposal of, 84

fatalities due to, 7–10
    pyrolysis of, 87
    toxic impurities in, 88
    use of, 6–13, 114
Pests (vertebrate), control of, 82
Pets, killed by pesticides, 82
Pharmacogenetics, 59–60
Pharmacokinetics, 15, 17, 25, 50, 88
Physico-chemical characteristics,
    toxicity and, 10, 111
Piscicides, assessment of, 43–45
    deliberate use of, 43, 83
Platt, Lord, opinion on LD$_{50}$, 4, 120
Populations, 6, 17, 45, 59, 119
Potentiation, definition of, 26
Primates (sub-human), in acute
    toxicology, 11
    skin penetration in, 105
Probit analysis, 19–23
Probits, see Probit analysis
Propellants, in aerosols, 111

Quantal response, definition of, 17
    polychotomous, 17

Re-entry time, after use of pesticides,
    106
Reptiles, toxicity of pesticides to, 45
Resistance to toxicants, 60
Respiratory tract, absorption from,
    107–111
    aspiration of vapours and fluids into,
    107
Response, age and, 51–56
    'all or none', 17
    extrapolation of, 14
    highly specific, 16
    interspecies variation in, 28–31
    'lethal synthesis', 16
    non-specific, 15
    polychotomous quantal, 17
    quantal, 17
    reactive, 15
    reproducibility of, 29
    sub-lethal, 14, 33
    subtle, 12, 14
    temperature and, 49, 63–67, 117
Risk–benefit analysis, 120
Routes (exposure), importance of,
    88–113

Safety, definition of, 3
Sex, hormone administration and, 59
    influence on acute response, 56–59

'metabolic body weight' and, 48
metabolism and, 57
rodents and, 57
sensitivity to intoxication, 56–59,
    116–117
Signs, of intoxications, 14
Skin, absorption through, 56, 94–106
'anti-transport' in, 97
appendages and penetration, 95–96
barrier zone in, 95
blood flow in, 100
diffusion through, 97, 99
epidermal thickness of, 99
exposure under occlusive conditions,
    104
macromolecules as penetrants of, 96
regional differences and penetrability
    of, 105–106
routes of penetration through, 95
species differences in penetrability, 38,
    104–105
Szakall layer in, 95
vapours as penetrants of, 103–104
Solvents, influence on acute toxicity,
    74–78
Species, availability for investigative
    toxicology, 34–45, 116
choice of for acute tests, 33–67, 104
extrapolation of findings between, 34,
    48, 50, 105
interactive effects in different, 28
types of in toxicology:
    amphibians, 45
    birds, 41
    fish, 43
    mammals, 35
    reptiles, 45
Statistical analysis, of acute data, 17–29
Stomach, absorption in, 89

Strain, effect of on response, 59–60
importance of in acute toxicology, 59–60
Stress, blood–brain barrier and, 62
caging and, 62
circadian rhythms and, 61
hibernation and, 63
infection and, 63
light and, 61, 63
physiological rhythms and, 60
temperature and, 63–67
Suicide, by misuse of pesticides, 81
Symptoms, of intoxication, 14
Synergism, definition of, 26, 74
interpretation of, 26
Synergists, use of in formulations, 79

Temperature, absorption and, 98
acute toxicity and, 49, 63–67, 117
poikilothermal animals and, 66
2,3,7,8-Tetrachlorodibenzo-p-dioxin, see
    Dioxins
Threshold limit, definition of, 3, 17
Time, as factor in acute toxicity, 22,
    70–71
integrated effect curves, 71
Toxicity, definition of, 1
'Toxicity index', definition of, 29
Transport, toxic hazard associated with,
    84

Vapours, skin penetration by, 103–104
Vehicle, absorption through skin and,
    101
bioavailability and, 74–78
definition of, 73
Viscosity, bioavailability and, 92
Vomit reflex, absence of in rodents, 92

Weather, cause of pesticide intoxication,
    86